ON THE SPECTRUM

An Autistic Look Into an Autistic Mind

Eric L David

On The Spectrum Copyright © 2021 by Eric L David. All Rights Reserved.

All rights reserved. No part of this book may be reproduced in any form or by any electronic or mechanical means including information storage and retrieval systems, without permission in writing from the author. The only exception is by a reviewer, who may quote short excerpts in a review.

Cover designed by Eric L David

This book is a work of fiction. Names, characters, places, and incicents either are products of the author's imagination or are used fictitiously. Any resemblance to actual persons, living or dead, events, or locales is entirely coincidental.

Visit my website at www.ericlynndavid.com

Printed in the United States of America

First Printing: Jan 2021

ISBN 9798590705863

Continuous improvement is better than delayed perfection.

—MARK TWAIN

We draw an ideological circle and those inside of it are thought of and treated differently from those outside of it.

—MAGUS PETER H GILMORE

I went to a bookstore and asked the saleswoman "where's the self-help section?" She said if she told me it would defeat the purpose.

—GEORGE CARLIN

This book is dedicated to the individual---for without the individual, freedom gets lost amongst the herd.

Contents

on the spectrum	1
SOCIAL INTERACTION	6
SENSORY OVERLOAD	80
ROUTINES, COMPULSIVENESS, AND RESTRICTED SPECIAL INTERESTS	126
FORMAL DIAGNOSIS	149
HOW I PERCEIVE THE WORLD	177
WORKS CITED	182
ABOUT THIS WORK	183

SOCIAL INTERACTION

The notion of autism has undergone several incarnations over the decades (since the 1940's).

The fact that I am currently writing about the subject doesn't surprise me even though I was late-diagnosed as an adult and completely slipped through the very few support systems we had in place while I was growing up. The fact that I'm writing---period---may surprise some folks who don't quite understand what this diagnosis is about. That is precisely why I'm doing this.

There are a few medical terms that need to be understood prior to going any further in this book so that the jargon doesn't get too confusing. I find most people who are not part of a specific field of study despise the jargon associated with that field. Keep in-mind that I am a technical professional, and my degrees are not in the medical or psychological fields. I simply have lifelong experience with this particular disorder and a special interest in its study.

Autism Spectrum Disorder (ASD) is a neurodevelopmental disorder that is defined by the American Psychiatric Association as a single continuum of mild to severe impairments in the two domains of social communication and restrictive repetitive behaviors/interests rather than being distinct disorders [1, p. xlii]. The baseline for this diagnosis is that it occurs within the first 3 to 5 years of childhood and continues through adulthood. There is no cure for autism. There is behavior therapy (communication, physical coordination, social introduction and continuous education), but for the core diagnosis, it remains a lifelong disorder.

The DSM-V also breaks ASD down into three severity levels [1, p. 52]:

Level 3 – Requiring Very Substantial Support

Level 2 – Requiring Substantial Support

Level 1 – Requiring Support (aka "High Functioning")

Other important definitions:

Hyperfocus – an accelerated state of attention that can consume a large portion of time and energy; the best comparison is to think of a cat. When a cat is focused on something, nothing can break its focus not even touch.

Hyper-Sensitivity – an intensified state of sensory acceleration that can be excessive and painful but is purely mental not physical. Lights can be too bright; sounds can be too loud; touch can be too aggravating; smell can be too atrocious. Often, being hyper-sensitive is an unpleasant experience.

Hypo-Sensitivity – a dulled state of sensory deceleration that can be near-numbing in effect. Touch, taste, smell, certain sights, and certain sounds can go unnoticed. Often, being hypo-sensitive can cause someone to seek out certain physical sensations or scents or lights, especially if repetitive and intense. Note: there is an overlap between hyperfocus and hypo-sensitivity in that being hyperfocused can dull certain senses during a specific activity or state of captured attention.

Meltdown – a common description for what is also known as an overwhelming situation. If senses are overloaded or specific circumstances/environmental factors are too intense, a person typically shuts-down/locks-up or "explodes" into a rage of emotion to release the build-up. A common reaction to someone who is feeling overwhelmed is flight or fight---intense anger or escape to a quiet, "safe" place to calm down. Sometimes, being overwhelmed triggers stimming.

Stimming – short for self-stimulating, this is an often-repetitive physical series of gestures (rocking back-and-forth, tapping fingers, finger snapping, lip biting, face rubbing, hair stroking/pulling, digging under the nails, foot tapping, hand "flapping," and a host of other coping mechanisms) that either bring a person UP out of a state of nervousness or boredom or bring a person DOWN from excitement or anxiety.

Coping Mechanism – any number of techniques or devices to help a person calm down/deal with anxiety or a stressful situation/environment. Some people turn to alcohol to help cope with social situations; some use drawing or video games or music with headphones to silence-out overwhelming noise. Some coping mechanisms can lead to addiction or strong dependency.

As an infant, we don't notice a difference. As a toddler, we still don't notice a difference. It's when we start school that we immediately notice we are different, but we don't know exactly why or how. Fortunately, there are a good number of screening tools and an early detection system in place that helps identify kids on The Spectrum (among other challenges) so that they may not have to endure what we adults---who had little-to-no tools or systems in place---have had to learn over the years. As an adult, a formal diagnosis is difficult, but it can still be challenging to identify in a young child. Adults learn how to adapt (or, at least, try to) and compensate.

We acquire/collect a repertoire of tricks to help us deal with the sensory overload; we develop or discover coping mechanisms and tools to help us deal with the social inadequacies and natural responses we were never born with in the first place. Some of us are fortunate enough to have a loving parent(s) or sibling or partner or friend to remind us of what we're doing right or wrong, no matter how trivial it may seem.

The most important takeaway is that being on The Spectrum does not mean mentally impaired or handicapped or impossible to work with or a means to giving up. Most humans are born with one or more challenges to overcome---some of which don't manifest until old age. ASD is simply one challenge, and it is a difficult one. A person who has learned how to work WITH it instead of AGAINST it has learned how to live with it and is a much stronger person as a result. Companies are learning (as of this writing) to specialize their hiring towards those who are on The Spectrum because they are starting to realize there are significant STRENGTHS that come with this disorder. There is a sense of intense concentration and focus, attention to specific detail, an adherence to following rules, and a unique way of looking at any situation from a perspective that most others are unaware of---all of these can only make a company stronger.

I'm fortunate in that I learned how to adapt to corporate rules and how to apply my strengths to any company I worked for to help them become more productive. I learned how to apply my strong sense of analytical and visual thinking to numerous projects and troubleshooting opportunities. I've climbed more than one corporate "ladder."

I'm fortunate that I continue striving for higher education degrees and training opportunities because I refuse to be held back by anything that I have control over. I've overcome significant challenges in school prior to college and stand as a testament that anything is possible with determination, alone. Skillsets are secondary.

Lastly, I'm immensely fortunate in that I was raised by a loving, caring family who accepted and supported me---and still do---I wouldn't trade my experiences with them for anything. My only regret is that I rarely discussed the items in this book with them when I was a kid, and I wish I could have written this book, put together my blog site, and gone through formal diagnosis back then.

Social Deficiencies

Socializing is something I have always struggled with---as do us all who are on The Spectrum. There are numerous reasons why it is a struggle, and each vary depending on the individual every bit as much as personality types may vary. Often, those of us on The Spectrum are perceived as just being very shy and quiet and reserved. Often, we are perceived as being geeky or nerdy. Sometimes, we are perceived as being somewhat creepy because we stare from a distance or listen-in on conversations not meant for us.

Sometimes, we just stand nearby without really interacting. These unusual behaviors are our way of interacting, socially. Still, there are some of us who are schizoid avoidant and have no desire to interact with another human being---ever. Thankfully, that is not my case. I actually want to interact, and I've had numerous failures in the past while attempting to do so. I've only recently shown significant progress participating in group conversations... only recently.

The DSM-V describes the Part A criteria as having persistent deficits in social communication and social interaction across multiple contexts, as manifested by the following, currently or by history [1]:

1. Deficits in social-emotional reciprocity, ranging, for example, from abnormal social approach and failure of normal back-and-forth conversation; to reduced sharing of interests, emotions, or affect; to failure to initiate or respond to social interactions.

2. Deficits in nonverbal communicative behaviors used for social interaction, ranging, for example, from poorly integrated verbal and nonverbal communication; to abnormalities in eye contact and body language or deficits in understanding and use of gestures: to a total lack of facial expressions and nonverbal communication.

3. Deficits in developing, maintaining, and understanding relationships, ranging, for example, from difficulties adjusting behavior to suit various social contexts; to difficulties in sharing imaginative play or in making friends; to absence of interest in peers.

Childhood

As infants, we don't know any better. We have nothing to compare against... nothing to cross-reference. What is good? What is bad? What is acceptable? What is achievement? What is the future? There is no past because it hasn't been written yet.

Imagine being born into a world without all of the natural adaptations most "normal" people are born with. Human beings are social creatures by natural design.

I've mentioned this several times, already, but home was safe. My social circle was at home. I didn't need outside friends. I had my toys, my movies, my music, and my family. What more could I have wanted? At some point, a parent will try to get a child to interact with other children. After all, it's a healthy thing. No one wants his/her child to be alone. It isn't healthy. It isn't natural.

There is a difference between being alone and loneliness, however.

I was never lonely. My every waking minute was occupied with something to do. I knew my grandparents were in another part of the house and often drifting from one part to the other or from inside to outside the house. My parents were around---even when they weren't (parents do need to go to work at some point; parents do need to go out and have fun at some point), it felt like they were always there. The times when Grandma babysat me, I really didn't require it (well, maybe for food), but my real babysitter was preoccupation with… everything.

After discussing it with Mom, and pulling from every memory I could, I don't believe I was all that abnormal acting when I was at home. I trusted the family. I don't believe there was anything terribly obvious that my parents or grandparents could have picked up on, behaviour-wise or eye contact-wise. Back then, there was no toddler testing. If a kid seemed healthy, so be it. Mental health was really non-existent as a concern. Would I have tested positive for autism back then under the old DSM manual? I would have been a tough case because there was no significant delay in speech.

I learned to speak and pronunciate just fine but had extreme difficulty controlling my pitch (which lasted well past my teens), sometimes sounding very high and sometimes sound very low. My speaking was more on the selective-mutism side because I would rattle-on at home but be mute anywhere else (unless my parents were right there with me). If someone spoke to me and tried to get me to reciprocate, I would go silent. My motor reflexes were normal, although I was quite clumsy and accident prone. I was also extremely sensitive when I was teething (most kids are), but I remember going through the pain to this very day.

Incidentally, I was born with a Simian Crease on my right hand, or what is now called Single Palmar Crease since it isn't as an offensive name, now ("simian" refers to an ape). A single palmar crease appears in about 1 out of 30 people. Males are twice as likely as females to have this condition. Some single palmar creases may indicate problems with development and be linked with certain disorders [2]. It's often associated with Down Syndrome, but there are also a host of other associative disorders---and, there are people who are perfectly neurotypical who have one.

There are some associations with autism, but scientific studies have proven having (or not having) a Single Palmar Crease is a poor indicator of autism. I simply found it fascinating that mine does correlate. The single line running across my entire right hand is the actual crease (below left photo). My left hand is quite normal, crease-wise (below right photo).

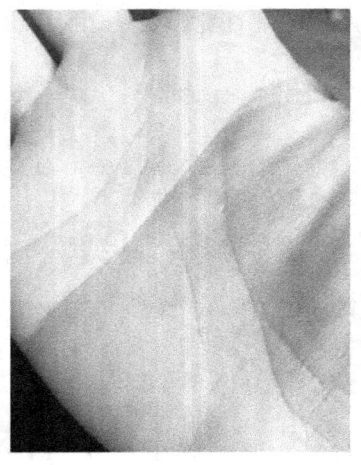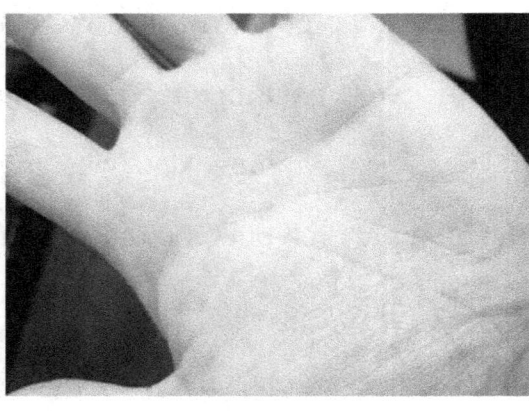

I did have a HELLUVA' time tying my shoes. I simply couldn't grasp the concept. I would stare at the intertwined loops that my parents had tied for me---for, I don't know how long. I would just stare at the shoestrings. I was bewildered by them. When I did have the opportunity to tie them on my own, I would build these shoestring towers that twisted up but didn't tie against anything. They'd spill over, and I'd trip and fall over them. Shoestrings were my nemeses when riding a bicycle (which I learned rather quickly---I was off of training wheels in just a couple of weeks) because they would always get wrapped around the pedals, and I'd go sailing over the handlebars and scrape my face in the dirt or asphalt. My knees were regularly skinned-up, and my parents were used to picking gravel out of my wounds. Pain didn't bother me. I wasn't afraid of getting hurt at all. I rarely felt the actual pain---it was the situation that would cause me to cry, sometimes.

The most important thing I can stress is that at home I was rarely unhappy or bored. I always entertained myself… always was fascinated by something. I surrounded myself with toys, music, and television. Nothing has changed to this day. My parents described me as a jovial, happy baby.

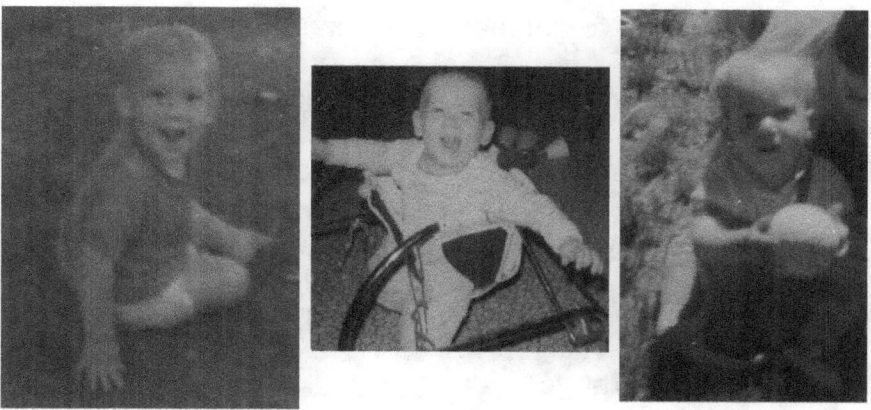

I loved animals, in particular. Grandma's home was like a miniature farm because she had a huge garden, chickens, a cow, dogs, cats, and even turkeys and geese. I spent a great deal of time outside in the very early years because my senses weren't really bothering me at that time. This is quite normal for those of us on The Spectrum because certain things don't really start manifesting until the first 5 years, depending on what they may be. When I was outside, I was plagued by bugs and getting things in my eyes, constantly falling and getting bruised and cut, and being chased by a mad turkey. The cow and the turkey freaked me out---so did the bugs---but it was a normal freak-out. Nothing really unusual. I had my intense brooding moments, but home was home---it was safe.

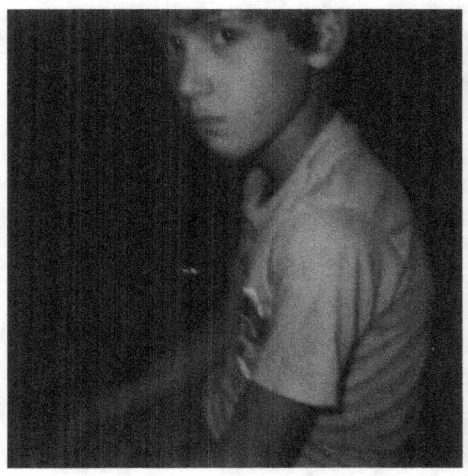

It wasn't until my parents tried to get me to socialize---to step out of the safety of home (which included the fenced front and back yards) and interact with other strange, noisy creatures called kids---that some things began to materialize. I didn't want to. I wanted to stay home. We had a fairly populated neighborhood with a lot of kids my age and a bit older, mixed races (a main reason why I have no comprehension of racism), and a mostly low-to-medium income range.

"We tried to get you to play with the other kids, but you never wanted to leave the house!" ~ Mom.

Every time I would see another kid, I would instantly lockup and go mute. My eyes would divert away (usually down and to one side), and the first opportunity there was to get away I would take it. I couldn't really understand anything the other kids were saying, implying, or doing. They weren't really as into the same things I was, for one thing. I wasn't really into sports, and they weren't into InfraMan™ or Micronauts™. They would be touchy and excitable... it was like they were speaking a different language when they tried to start a conversation of some kind. Girls were even worse!

I did have a very special "friend" that was a stuffed dog I named Preshy. I don't know where I got the name from, but I suspect it was short for "precious." The name and circumstance, alone, begs one to think of J.R.R. Tolkien's literary character, Gollum™, who referred to The One Ring as "my precious." I hadn't watched the cartoon, yet, by that point, so this was entirely coincidental. I carried Preshy everywhere I went---by the neck---until his body separated from his head, but I didn't care. It ended up being so dirty and eaten away that Mom had to throw it away without my knowing about it. I was deeply upset when I found out.

When Mom bought him for me at a rummage sale, he was intact. His ears and tail were mostly felt. He had a triangular, pink felt tongue. His ears, tail, and limbs were stitched with yarn to his body. His eyes were black marbles. His nose was a very hard black plastic. He had lighter felt eyebrows that gave him a worried look (I interpreted it as a worried look – it might have been friendly for all I could tell). I gripped him by the throat for years---hardly ever parted with him for more than a few minutes. Eventually, the stuffing wore-out where I gripped him, and the weight of his body tore the material holding his neck to his body together. When the head separated, fully, I was not concerned about it. I kept his head with me for months after that, still holding him by the neck.

Below, are two illustrations of Preshy (the closest I can recall – he was actually quite the ugly stuffed dog, but I loved him) with the left looking much like he was when I first received him; the right image is how he ended up (bodiless):

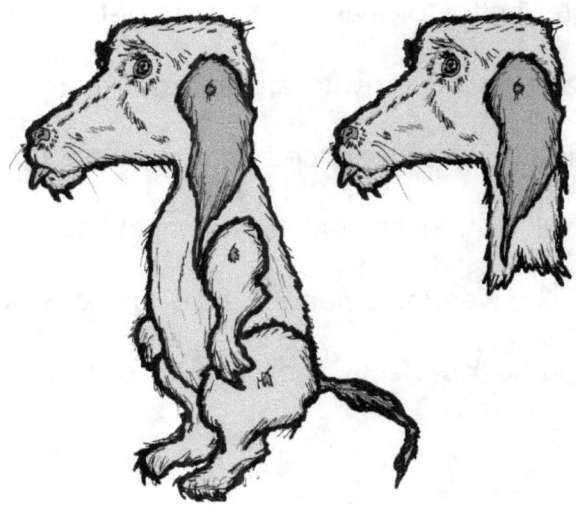

Around the 5-year mark, I started becoming hypersensitive to touch. The wind started really bothering me… blowing my hair (ref. the Sensory Overload chapter), causing me to scratch my head and even pull chunks of hair out. At the time, I didn't realize it was the wind blowing my hair strands. I simply thought I was feeling something crawling in my hair each time I went outside. It took me some time to make the correlation. Even so, I would still go outside.

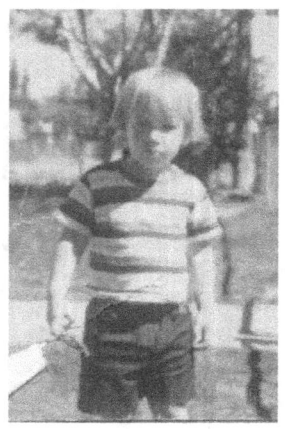

I started getting earaches---mainly in my left ear. I hated wearing hats or ski caps or hoods of any kind, so I had no protection for my ears. Mom would try to get me to wear something, but I would just take it right off. I remember many nights in the winter where I had to sleep on a hot water bottle to heal my earache of-the-month. At one point, I had an earache so bad that I ended up with a perforated eardrum (torn eardrum), and the pain was unlike anything I had experienced prior to that point and for quite some time after. I was fortunate that it eventually healed (took about 1 month, and the doctor was expecting me to eventually be wearing a hearing aid). One day, it simply healed, and the pain was gone, and I could hear perfectly fine.

I would play with Grandpa's hand tools inside his toolshed, and the pliers and vice grips looked like dinosaurs to me. I would give them their own language and let them talk to one another with it. I remember looking up at Mom, once, and she was staring down at me while I was using that made up language---I think it sort of creeped her out because it really did sound like a foreign language of some kind. I instantly became self-conscious and stopped the activity and moved on to something else.

At times, I my cousins, aunts and uncles came over to visit Grandma. My cousin, Mike, was the closest thing to a brother I ever had. He was extremely controlling, loud, physically abrasive, and not exactly a good influence, but he loved me very much. My aunts and uncles were absolutely terrifying. They were LOUD, and their voices hurt my ears. They were intimidating, and they would order me to come to them (because I tried to hide from them), and they couldn't understand why I was so quiet around them---why I didn't really want to have anything to do with them. I knew why, but I couldn't tell them why. I would go mute and stiff every time. The most common comment I heard from them: "why are you so skinny?!!! Look. He's so skinny!"

To be honest, I really didn't know whether I was skinny or not because I never really paid attention to my reflection in the mirror except for necessary toiletries. I had a bowl haircut. I wore whatever clothes happened to be given me. I didn't care how dirty or clean I was at any given time (ref. Sensory Overload chapter regarding my hatred of showers and baths).

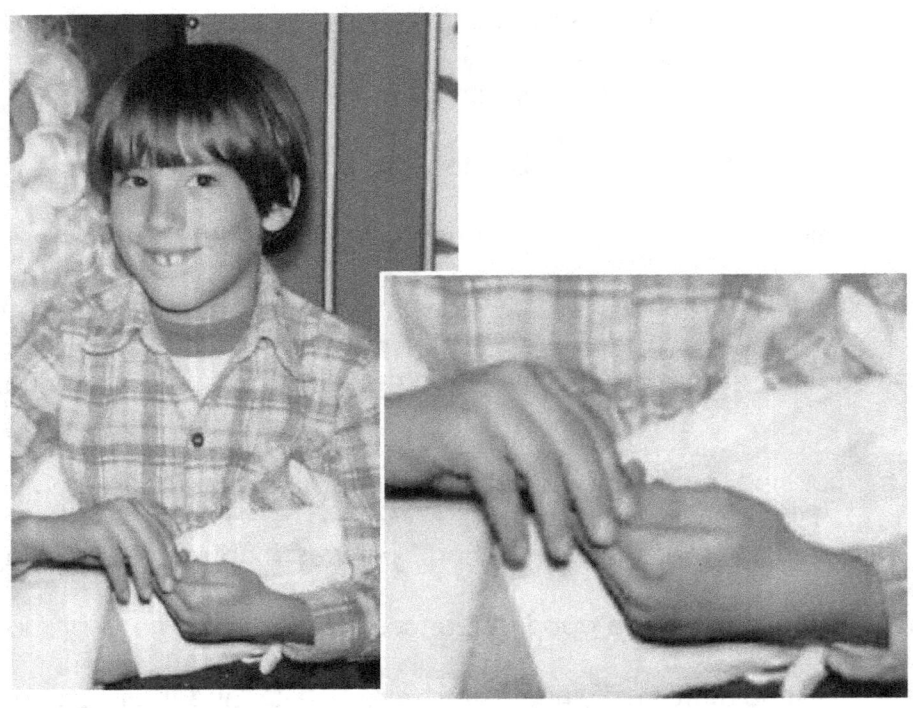

Santa Claus was very important to me, and I continued believing in him until the 6th Grade. I remember being told the story of this magical person somewhere between 1 and 3 years-old, and my parents bought me several vinyl albums that I would play, continuously, from the end of November through December. My parents took me to see Santa at the mall, and I was thrilled and terrified at the same time. I was perfectly fine standing near him, but the moment they put me on his lap, and he held onto me, I lost it. I locked-up at first then burst out in tears afterwards.

It took me a few years to get used to being held by Santa. If you look closely at the photo above, you can see me stimming (self-stimulating) with my fingers. This was a typical nervous reaction I would engage in. I would dig under my nails, repetitively. Even at that particular point, I was still apprehensive about being touched. Regardless, Christmas and Santa Claus were highlights of my life, and I have nothing but very pleasant memories. I believe this is why I still love and celebrate Christmas and am still devoted to my large collection of Christmas music.

During these years, my family was heavily involved with Church. We would go Sundays and Wednesdays. Because I was a bit more… mature… than the other kids in Church, I went to only one Sunday School session (geared for kids and focused more on Bible stories). Our family read the King James Bible for years before that, so I already had Revelations and Isaiah and Psalms and… memorized. Sunday School was terribly boring.

I insisted on sitting in the regular congregation. Unfortunately, our pastor singled me and another kid out by making us stand up in front of the congregation and sing---SING---"This Little Light of Mine." I… went… stiff. I kept my head down, eyes down, and mumbled while the other boy sang more loudly. I was… enraged and humiliated. My parents knew what was happening to me and pulled me back down in the pew. A few months later, my parents thought it would be a healthy thing for me to go to Church Camp. I was opposed to it, but they knew how introverted I was and that this experience might help me make friends---socialize---maybe get out of my "shell." This was a mistake, but I cannot blame my parents for trying. I rode in one of the church vans with older kids (2 of which couldn't keep their hands off of each other) up to… wherever the hell that camp was… in the mountains, somewhere outside of town.

The gastrointestinal issues kicked-in (more on that, later), but I was able to be discreet. I never took a shower until the end of the week---when our pastor insisted I take one. We all slept in bunk beds in the same cabin---about 8 of us. One day, I was trying to explain… something… I was having an issue with and the pastor kept yelling at me to "shut up!" to "shhhh!" The other boys could talk, but he insisted I stay silent. I don't know why. I'll never understand that situation or how I made him so angry at me.

There was a kind of prom at the end of the week, and the camp had us kids all do a kind of runway show… girls and boys… and we were supposed to walk out there and get judged by the crowd as to how "cute" we were. It's quite disturbing thinking about it, now. There were more attractive boys ahead of me, and the girls would howl at them as they passed by on the stage.

When it was my turn to walk out---I fast-walked---had a huge grin on my face the entire time, eyes downcast---and got the hell off the stage. There was only silence---no howling for me. That made my self-confidence FAR worse than it was. One girl came up to two of us standing outside the cabin, and the boy asked me if I wanted him to ask her if she wanted to go to Camp Prom. I shook my head up-and-down (yes). He asked her. She shouted: "YUCK!!!" He, then, asked her if she would go with HIM, instead ("well, would you go with me, then?"). She became bashful, instantly, and said: "yes." All of this occurred in front of me. Again… not good for my self-confidence.

I became as reclusive as I could for the remainder of my stay in that place and played tetherball during the day---no one else required---just me. We finally left that place, and when we got back into town, my parents were there to pick me up at the church. I couldn't get in the car fast enough. I just wanted to go home. They asked me how Camp was, and I told them everything. They promised to never make me do something like that ever again. They were starting to understand.

When we talk about empathy deficiencies, an example would be my one childhood friend (for 2 years), Donald. He was a very emotional, expressive person. I didn't understand how important our friendship actually was to him until the day our family moved from the neighborhood to a different part of the city. One day I was there; the next day, I was gone. It never occurred to me to even let him know. It never occurred to me to leave a phone number or something. In my absolutist mind, he would understand because I was no longer there. It was logical. Somehow, one day, he managed to get hold of me with a letter in the mail---it was a very sad letter where he was upset why I didn't tell him that we were leaving. I couldn't understand why he was sad about it. This is how the autistic mind works, socially. In psychological terms, it's called schizoid personality type (somewhat avoidant). No wonder we struggle.

If the friendship ended when I was aware it would, I was perfectly fine with it. If the friendship ended when I was NOT aware it would, I would slip into a deep sadness---well, depression, actually. This goes back to the need for control. We need to control our lives and environments so that everything is predictable.

Anything expected that's on our terms is perfectly acceptable; anything unexpected that's not on our terms, is not acceptable, and we lose it---instant meltdown of some kind. Again, my tantrums at the toddler stage turned into lockups during the pre-adolescent and adolescent stages---and persist as such to this very adult stage.

I did have one friend for a few years whom I would visit about once-per-month. He lived several neighborhoods away, so my parents or Grandma would take me to his house, and they would visit with his parents while the two of us socialized. He was much like me but even more introverted than I was. We basically exchanged comments and talked AT one another rather than really engaging in conversation. We would compare our toys, but there really wasn't a typical interaction as one might expect between boys at a young age. I suspect he, too, was on The Spectrum.

I accompanied Mom to where she worked, sometimes, and there was a Kenpo Karate instructor who was a customer. He looked at me and suggested I come by his Karate school and start training. I just did my typical big smile and said nothing. He would come back once-per-week, and I would hide in the bathroom before he would see me so that I didn't have to endure his repeated invites. I wasn't afraid of him or creeped-out by him, by any means. It was the thought of going to a school and physically interacting with other people that terrified me.

My family moved around the city a lot. We averaged 2.2 years per-residence across 15 different residences (mostly apartments or town houses). None of this was my doing. I would've been perfectly content staying put in one location because, once I took up roots, I was content---by that point, we'd end up moving again. Most of this was my dad's doing. He would get bored and wanted to move, I suppose.

An incident occurred while I was riding a city bus to school. A frequent passenger, whom I recognized, an elderly woman, looked at me while I was standing up from my seat and said: "my, you're getting quite tall." I didn't acknowledge her. I didn't know how to answer her. It was a statement… a comment. Do I say "thank you"? Do I say "yes. I am"? In my mind, she was stating something obvious, and there was no point in me saying anything further. I simply walked off the bus and went on about my business. This particular incident---I label an incident---because it was an example of how difficult conversation was for me, especially since I was interacting more with strangers during this time period. At the same time, I feel as though it was a missed opportunity to make an elderly lady feel... better... about making what I know now to be a compliment. I feel... bad... about it.

One day my paternal step-grandfather decided to pick me up to go fishing for the weekend with his friends and their kids. I did NOT want to go, but my parents coaxed me into it. I barely said a word the entire time. I remember asking one pointless question in an attempt to start a conversation, but that was a failed attempt. The other boys did all of the talking, and I just stayed nearby and listened. I went into the lake with the rest of the kids, once, and stayed in there for too long (was wading the entire time because I really wasn't a good swimmer---still not to this day)... I guess I was in another hyperfocus state because I wasn't aware that I was cold.

When I finally came out of the water, I was shaking, heavily. The adults were concerned I was going into shock/hypothermia. They were getting very concerned, actually. They put me in the camper bed with a bunch of warm blankets, and the shaking finally went away after about 20 or 30 minutes. I was happy to go home, but I did enjoy the thought of spending some time with a step-grandfather I barely knew.

School

One day, something horrific happened. My parents took me to something called kindergarten. School. My world was rocked, and not in a good way. I will mention many times that home was safe throughout this book. School and going out in public, on the other hand---not so much. I was 5 years-old when I started school. At that time, I was 1 year younger than my peers (6 years-old was the typical starting age for kindergarten). My parents felt I was intelligent enough to start early. I learned how to read, write, and learned basic arithmetic because they taught me ahead-of-time. They were quite confident in my intellect.

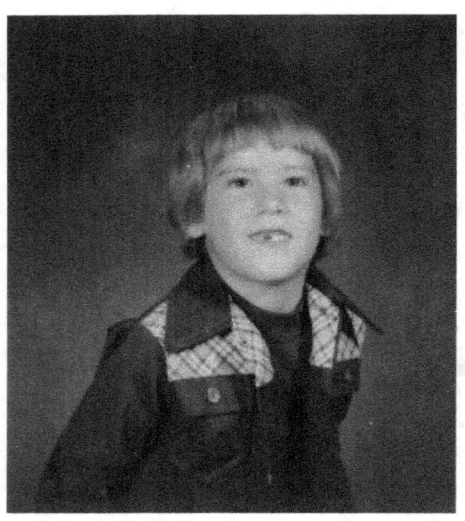

My first day of kindergarten was… strange. I didn't have a meltdown like some kids might have. I simply retreated inside myself. I needed to understand why I was there and not home. Who were these rowdy kids on the other side of the room? Why were they looking at me? I didn't want to go over there where they were at. It was best to stay standing near the corner and study the room. It was best to look for things I was familiar with, instead; otherwise, this was a pretty damned boring experience and served no purpose.

The classroom, itself, was interesting. It was two conjoined metal barracks (army barracks, perhaps) with the main class area in the front and physical activity area in the back. A mini library was on the far side, and a science area (with aquariums) was near the window-side.

I noticed the bookshelves, first, and gravitated toward them. There were objects on the shelves that I was familiar with. Something... relatable... something... safe: dinosaurs and books! I stood in the center of both shelves and stared at the contents, feeling quite elated at this point. I knew it was impolite to just reach out and touch things that were not mine, so I walked up to both adults in the room (the teacher and her assistant) and actually spoke for the very first time while having been in the room for... I really don't know how long. I asked very politely: "can I pick up one of the dinosaurs?"

My teacher said: "well, yes."

I darted over to the shelf and took the Triceratops (my favourite dinosaur) off the shelf and sat down on the floor with it. I looked up at the Tyrannosaurus Rex, got up from the floor, walked over to the teacher and politely asked if I could pick up the other dinosaur. Again, she said I could. I repeated the process but had both dinosaurs on the floor with me at this point. I wasn't that interested in the Brachiosaurus or Stegosaurus or Pterodactyl toys. I had the two I cared about. I wasn't really playing with them, per se'. I was just looking them over, admiring their quality because they were great looking, and lifelike toys.

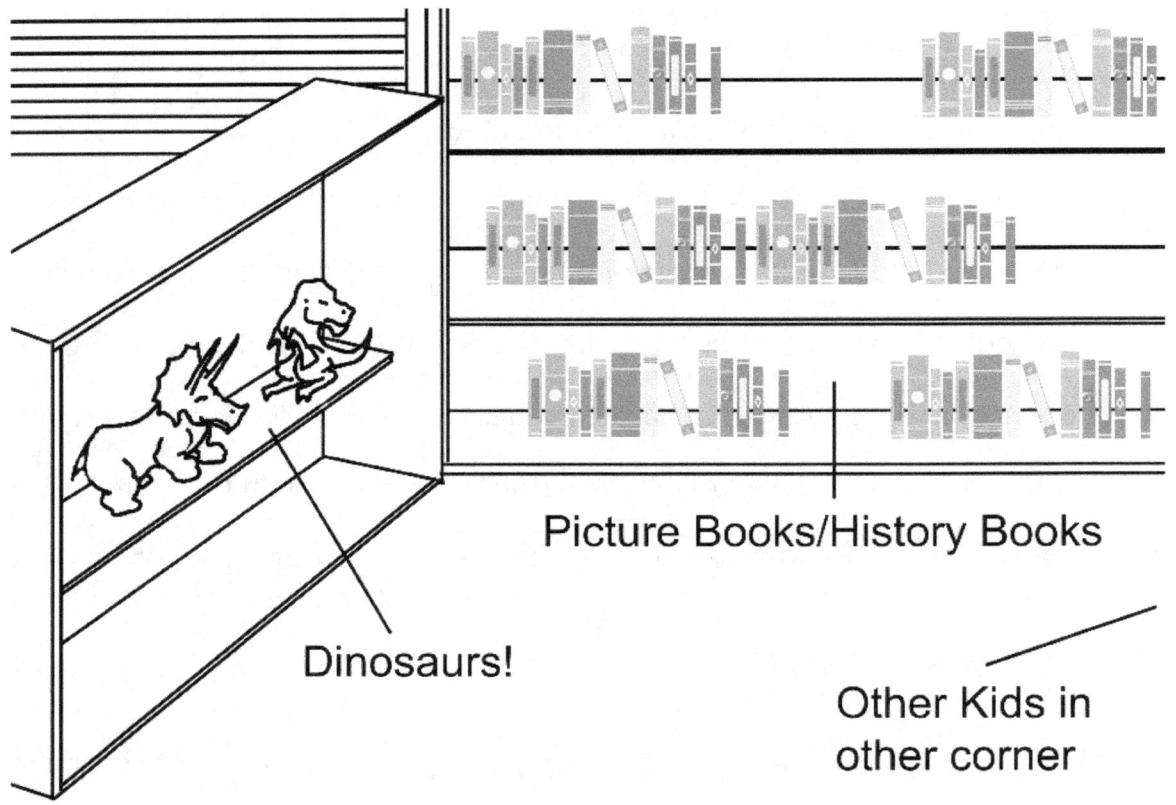

I would describe my kindergarten teacher and her evil assistant as mean and intolerant human beings not fitting to be teaching anyone much less children (yes, I do remember their names, but I'm purposely not listing them). They didn't have the patience or personality. I will say, however, that my teacher knew when something wasn't quite right with a student.

When she noticed I was not socializing with the other children and was taken-back by how formal and polite I was about asking to play with the toys on the shelves--- when I actually did speak, she had me moved into a Special Education class. She knew something wasn't quite normal with me but didn't know what to do with me. I wasn't interested in intermingling with the other kids---they were uninteresting and noisy and far too excited.

I was in the special education class for 1 week. They didn't teach me the things my parents already had. Instead, I and about 4 other kids were given cutouts (mine was a grasshopper) to color with crayons and other visual activities---incredibly boring and unchallenging. I never told my parents. It wasn't until a Friday that my parents asked the right question that triggered a specific response, and I was able to tell them that I wasn't in my regular class anymore, that I was in a different class, and I showed them my colored-in grasshopper.

My parents were irate and confronted my teacher and explained to her that I already knew how to write, do math, and read. I was in the room at the time, exploring the desks in the room but listening quite intently to the conversation. My teacher was trying to make the case for me to stay 1 year behind because I started too early---she really didn't know what the difference in me was, but she knew there was something different. My parents convinced her (rather assertively with some interspersed colorful metaphors) that I was smart enough to remain in this grade at my age and in this level of class and not be in a Special Education class. From that moment-on, I was treated differently by my teacher and her assistant. The assistant, in particular, would ostracize me from some of the group activities and have me read some of the picture books in the corner of the room. I didn't understand the difference and simply complied. I didn't know any better.

Because the schools I attended were not equipped to diagnose children for most psychological disorders beyond more traditional learning disabilities and "handicaps," they had me tested for what they could They assumed there was something wrong with me but didn't know what, so they regularly tested my hearing. I went from kindergarten through 2nd grade (first 3 years of school) having my hearing tested on a monthly basis.

I would sit in a chair with these huge headphones on my head. The tester would step out of the room and ask me to raise either my left or right hand, depending on which side of the headphones I would hear very high and very low pulse sounds. My hearing was excellent (too good, in some ways), and I passed their tests, but they continued testing me, anyway. I never thought to question this because I thought it was something that all kids at school went through. Once again, I never told my parents until they asked the right question one day, and I was able to tell them about the hearing tests. My parents complained to the school, but nothing really changed. It wasn't until we moved, and I started 3rd Grade at a different school, that the hearing tests stopped. I'm assuming the health transcripts did not transfer with me.

Below, is a summary of my first 3 years:

Kindergarten. I did not like the teacher and her assistant. They both treated me differently (I interpreted it as "mean") after they tried putting me in a Special Education class for 1 week. I tolerated my classmates. My first kiss by a girl happened here, and I freaked-out/ran away after she kissed me. The other kids were laughing. She wasn't. I think I hurt her feeling by my reaction.

1st Grade. I Loved my teacher. Mrs. Schulz. My fellow students were the same from kindergarten, so they were familiar to me. I would spend days staring at their faces and their hair so that I could try to recognize them, later on. She introduced us to ART, DANCE, SPANISH and MUSIC with guest teachers. The guest art teacher taught me to never erase my mistakes but to build on them. Music class was awkward because the other kids would run up and take the good instruments, so I was stuck with a tambourine, a triangle, or maracas. No one wanted to dance with me (the girls were repulsed by me for some reason). One girl even said: "yuck!" We went on field trips, and I would lose control of my "bodily functions" every single time we'd leave for a trip---it was a change of environment and schedule, and my little mind couldn't handle it, and my body would react. I came home, many nights, with the "unfortunate results," and Mom couldn't understand why---what was causing it. I was unable to explain why. I would stay silent and be angry (kicked a hole in Grandma's back door once because I was so mad at myself and the situation).

2nd Grade. I liked my teacher, but she was physically abusive. Mrs. Salisbury. She spanked me in front of the class because I couldn't understand one of the assignments and went up to ask her to explain it. This same teacher picked me up and slammed me down on the cafeteria bench because I wouldn't eat my sweet potatoes. I was spanked by my Physical Education teacher, Mr. Children (or Childers or Childress). I never knew what I did wrong, but he asked me to come up in front of the class, turn around, touch my toes—and WHAP! He spanked me so hard that I took several big steps forward and almost fell on my face. The rest of the class laughed. I was embarrassed and confused and just remained silent as usual. During a soccer match, I scored for the opposing team because I didn't understand which way to go… what the rules were… didn't understand… just knew I could run really FAST and had control of the ball. All of the kids laughed at me. From that point-on, I was told to clean up the sports closet and not allowed to play any sports or be on any teams.

Home was my sanctuary because it was safe. I had a loving, caring, understanding family who didn't consider me any less than anyone else---they simply thought I was forever shy and very into the things I loved (toys, movies, music, drawing). I found school to be traumatizing and intolerable, but I had to endure it. I was bullied quite often, both emotionally and physically from fellow students to a handful of teachers.

I was mostly mute through the first eleven years with only a few forced exceptions. No one could comprehend what it was like suffering from sensory overload to social awkwardness to the effects of isolation for a child growing up in a public school system. Relationships were quite sparse, but I did have them. There would be that one close friend for a year or two---that was it. I never had a girlfriend in school, and it wasn't until 2003 that I actually started dating someone.

Friendships were hard to come by for me. I wanted to be part of a group, but I could never initiate anything, and if I were standing or assigned to a group in class, I was still very much my own person and did my own thing within it. Anyone who came into my life had to initiate it---I never made the first move---not ever. If someone was interested in speaking or sharing something with me, then, I surmised, that person must be worth keeping around. In a way, my avoidance and lack of approach was a kind of filter. It's possible I was turning a social handicap into a coping mechanism by turning my "shyness" into a screening mechanism. Either way, it was an unhealthy behaviour.

That one friend I would have, each year (they seemed to only last 1 year, but a lot of that was due to our relocating around the city), is someone I would just attach to only on the playground. In my mind, there was no room for more than 1 friend, so that was it. He was my friend, so that meant I must follow him everywhere he goes---I must learn from him and even try to imitate him (laughter, in particular, was something I tried to mimic). I would let him do the majority of the speaking, and I would either reciprocate with basic "yes" "yeah" "oh" "no" or a slight giggle. Once back in the classroom, however, I was in "class mode" and had no use for that friend.

Gastrointestinal issues plague autistic folks for various reasons and at varying levels of intensity and frequency of occurrence. For me, my issues started on Day One of school and continued. I believe a great deal of it is stress-induced in that the whole body simply locks-up, causing numerous issues. If the body can't do its natural processing job, then a host of issues will occur.

When I was younger, I simply would "lose control" of my bodily functions. It was immensely embarrassing, and my poor parents had no idea why I was that way. A kid like me is incapable of fully explaining what's causing it---can't explain that going out of a routine or comfortable "safe" and predictable environment causes a tremendous amount of stress on the mind and body. To this day, traveling (taking trips of any duration) causes a total body "lockup." Again, this is quite common for those of us on The Spectrum.

Here is a summary of the next 3 years of school (3rd Grade to 5th Grade):

3rd Grade. Absolutely terrified of this teacher (name omitted). He had a loud, abrasive voice. He was mean (not just to me). He wouldn't let me leave the room to go to the restroom, so I peed on my desk and all over the floor. He made me clean it up, afterward. This did NOT set well with my fellow students, and I was even more ostracized from them, socially. I did have 1 or 2 sort-of friends on the playground for a brief period of time. I accidentally turned on 1 of them and put him in a headlock in front of a small group of kids (after shouting "there he is! Let's go get him!"). After I let him go (didn't hurt him), he was crying and shouted "I HATE you!". I couldn't understand why he was mad at me. I was playing.

4th Grade. Loved my teacher. Mr. Marroquin. He was patient, caring, and a good teacher. He knew I was different from the other kids in class, and he would let me take books home from his library and let me keep several of them (which I still have). 1 friend, Arthur Young, took me under his wing and introduced me to the Herge' TinTin™ books---which I still read to this day. I received a Good Citizenship Award in 4th Grade – didn't know what it was for at the time just accepted it/had picture taken – still have it – years later I researched what the award was for: a citizenship award is given to students who exemplify superior honor and discipline within the classroom environment. Okay... well, I was silent and did what I was told and did my homework.

5th Grade. Loved my teacher. Mrs. Smith. She was a traditional education-driven teacher, but she was also approachable. I was bullied by several kids on the playground (held my head down on one of the big tires we had in the playground and wouldn't let me up). I told Mrs. Smith about it, but she told me "oh, no one held your head down, Eric…"). My first public speaking in front of a class happened here, and I used to almost pass-out or run out of the classroom and throw-up before or afterwards. Bullying incident 1) while standing in the cafeteria line, a boy came up and slugged me in the stomach… for no reason… knocked the air out of me; 2) boy on playground came up to me and started a fight… with us rolling along the ground---I remembered a self-defense technique Dad showed me and clawed his stomach to force him off of me---a teacher showed up and broke us apart---I will never know why that happened as I was just by myself… silent.

Our family moved to another part of the city, and I started a new school. It was terrifying enough to transition from Elementary School to Middle School because, now, I had to deal with more than one teacher, more than one class/subject, and far more faces, inconsistent seating arrangements, and a whole new school layout. All of these things are overwhelming to the autistic mind. Combine all of that with 4 bullying incidents in the 6th Grade, alone, and you have a very unhappy kid at school.

I found the kids in middle school were far more aggressive and singled-out anyone who was different from what they were already accustomed to. Perhaps, they were frustrated at their own change of environment and only knew how to take that frustration out on others.

Another example would be a fellow student named Nathan, who was physically challenged and was in a wheelchair. I watched a kid push Nathan (while in his wheelchair) down a ramp inside the school. He and his friends thought it was funny.

Nathan could have been injured, but he was quick-thinking and hit his right wheel break and banked right through some open doors, avoiding a collision with a wall that was in front of him.

Here is a summary of the next 3 years of school (6th Grade through 8th Grade):

6th Grade. Bullying incident 1) group of boys surrounded me in one of the school courtyards, knocked my books out of my hands, took my pen, and shoved me back-and-forth from one-to-another for no reason; 2) boy in locker room put me in a headlock and held me there for several seconds for no reason; 3) boy in gym class regularly picked on me verbally and physically---grabbed my nose many times, put me in a headlock, called me names, teased me about my appearance and clothes; 4) boy in class room teased me because I brought a comic book with me to class, and he said I was "a girl" and "a baby" because I was "still reading comic books." His friends all laughed at me, and he took the comic out of my hands and threw it on the floor and walked out. I was 30lbs underweight and weighed 60lbs compared to the other boys who weighed an average of 90lbs. Random muscle/joint pains became noticeable during this year and continued ever since.

7th-8th Grades. We moved to another part of the city, again, and I started another new school. Overall, my experience with this school was far more pleasant. I was able to talk to a few other kids, here. Most of the population was mixed race, and I found the minority students were far less abusive and exclusive than the predominately-non-minority kids were at my previous schools. I had only 1 bullying incident that occurred on the school bus with a kid who took a disliking towards me for some reason-

--I was mostly mute, so it certainly wasn't anything I said. I finally grew tired of his teasing and told him to meet me at the next bus stop; I stood there, waiting, but he never stepped off of the bus---he looked out the window, pointed at me, and laughed. From that point-on, he never messed with me. I spilt chocolate milk all over a girl in the cafeteria because I was so hyperfocused on standing up and putting my coat on correctly that I was no longer aware the milk was in my left hand---it gushed out all over her. I did not react. I was paralyzed. I just stood there while she was gasping. Another boy said something negative at me, grabbed up some napkins, and started drying her off. I left the area and went on about my business as if nothing happened. The girl who said "YUCK!" about me during Church Camp a few years prior was in my English class---I guess I was no longer as unattractive to her as I was back then, and I don't believe she remembered me from that incident, because she asked her friend to tell me that "she thinks you're cute." I simply kept working on my assignment and ignored both of them (not out of spite, mind you; this was out of… my aloofness back then).

High school is challenging all on its own, but for the autistic student, it's intimidating and overwhelming. I started high school while we were still living in the same home (as middle school), so I recognized a small number of the same kids I went to school with, previously. I hated this high school, in particular. The layout was archaic and inconsistent. I was forever getting lost because it took me much longer to get a routine down---was very difficult to memorize the layout.

I was mostly mute upon entering high school. I knew a couple of people (including my cousin), and I tried clinging to them, but they didn't want someone as naïve as I was being with them---they were concerned about corrupting me. My cousin said to me once: "you're a good guy. I'm a bad influence. I don't want to be a bad influence on you." Naturally, I couldn't comprehend this, and I was quite devastated. My only "hook" into the social community was erased.

I spent my days in-between classes alone. I would be on a bench by where the school buses dropped-off/picked-up (I believe it was my way of wanting to be as close to a method of escape as possible). I would sit on the bench with my headphones on, listening to music. No one came near me.

While in class, I did my damnedest to stay in the very back of the classroom. Typically, I would sit in the back LEFT corners. The only times I sat in the middle, center, or front desks was when the teacher assigned seats. Some teachers have no idea how horrific that is for us---we don't want to be forced to do something that takes us out of our comfort zone, and forcing us to sit in an uncomfortable part of the room will do that very thing. When I was forced to sit in those other areas of a classroom, I was stiff as a board and rarely turned around. I was mute. I was paralyzed.

Another factor in my choosing where to sit in a classroom had to do with the air vents and window positioning. Most of the schools I went to had very high, small windows that allowed enough daylight in the room to masque the morgue-like feeling classrooms self-imposed, so having to avoid the bright sunlight from a window wasn't too big of a chore. Avoiding air vents in a classroom, on the other hand, could sometimes be quite challenging and sometimes impossible. I would be miserable during summer anytime the cool air kicked-on and blew against my skin (ref. Sensory Overload chapter).

During my 9th Grade timeframe, I attempted to say hello to a lady who regularly passed in front of our home while on the way to the city bus stop. I had passed her numerous times, and it seemed like a good enough time to say "hi" and practice being cordial. She said nothing and ignored me as though I was not there. I told myself I would never initiate a "hi" attempt to someone ever again---he/she would have to say "hi" first. That's been my rule ever since.

My Spanish teacher once ask me why I was so quiet, why I didn't talk to anyone. I avoided eye contact much more, back then, so I just quick-glanced towards her and forced the words out: "to avoid my enemies." Her response: "oh, you don't have any enemies." I didn't respond. In my mind, I was constantly under attack (of some kind) every time I went to school. When you couple my past poor experiences with an unpredictable environment, I would go into survival mode... and, it showed.

Below, is the summary from my high school experiences:

9th Grade. Started high school but lasted only about 6 months before we moved to another part of the city... again. I finished my remaining 4 years at another high school. This particular high school I liked very much---it was easy to navigate (octagonal shaped center with peripheral buildings outside), the students seemed much less aggressive. I spent this entire year by myself and mostly mute. The only bullying I would experience was from the previous first high school experience, and it simply stopped from this point-forward. I had to adjust my learning method, this year, as I was struggling with tests, and my grades were average C's at best. Physical Education class sucked. While playing a team-based field Frisbee game, I intercepted the Frisbee for our team, and an opposing player became agitated and threw me to the ground---my team yelled at him, and he apologized. I didn't really get upset about the act as I had done my job---I actually caught that damned Frisbee! I did have difficulty figuring out how to stack the Frisbees inside their canister while two other students were helping---it was like a brain lock, and I didn't want to embarrass myself over such a simple task---one of the students: "come on, dude… just put them inside…"

10th Grade. I grew so tired of dealing with the anxiety of speaking in front of classes that I purposely ditched class whenever there was a speech day. I would take a zero for that portion of the assignment. I didn't care. At least, I found a way of getting away from it. I fell in love with my Reading teacher's handwriting style. I never saw capital letters like that before. I would imitate her style until it became my own (years later, I was told it was 18th Century Old English---but it wasn't mine---it was hers). I was still struggling adjusting to tests and an increase in homework, but I was better this year than last.

11th Grade. This was a great year---probably my favourite year of them all. It seemed like everything was in order and balanced. I discovered leather jackets, started working out more and building a little muscle, and discovered I was quite good in Creating Writing and History. It was here that I met my friend, Aaron (still friends to this day). He was a bit of an outcast, too, but he was far more self-confident and filled with high energy---a bit rowdy, but he took me in, and we were best friends at that point. He coaxed me out of the house and talked me into going to the show and hanging-out at the malls. We had a few fun, simple adventures. My grades were average B's and low A's, as I was finally adapting to high school earning/testing methods.

12th Grade. My grades were still easy A's and B's because I didn't really feel challenged enough to try too hard. I was lazy and coasted through my senior year. I helped give the answers to a World History test in class, one day. While the teacher stepped out of the class room, one of the students asked what the answer was to 1 of the questions, and immediately I blurted-out the answer... another student asked what the answer was to another question... I answered, again... then another... and another... the entire class ACED their test that day. I contributed several illustrations, 1 poem, and 1 short story to our high school literary book and was quite proud of them (still have a copy)---also contributed a drawing of a knight to our yearbook. There was absolutely no way I was going to ask anyone to the prom. There was no one to ask, for that matter. I still felt a bit insecure about my appearance and felt too unattractive to talk to anyone. I was so happy to graduate and get away from public school. It was like leaving prison, I suppose. I didn't want to go to my graduation ceremony, however, but the school forced us all to endure it. I was still quite uncoordinated and messed-up the handshake procedure during my graduation ceremony---the principal handed the diploma to my left hand and extended his right, but I crisscrossed hands and grabbed the diploma with my right and tried to shake his hand with my left. The most common comment I heard was "you're that guy who draws all the time."

During my 11th and 12th grade years, the muscle/skeletal pains were at their worst. I would get off of the school bus, and would be limping halfway home due to sudden, sharp pains in my hips (sometimes, it would be the knees). There were some days I had to sit on one of the park benches halfway home. The muscle pains would hit mostly after school and rarely during school. It was a very delayed reaction that I could not explain. I blamed the pain on improper warming-up before I would practice martial arts, but that wasn't the issue. The psychosomatic effects of anxiety were the source of my pain.

I didn't understand how much impact the mind had on the body and that, each time I would enter a stressful environment or situation, it was the mind's equivalent to entering a war zone of some kind---the body's natural response of flight-or-fight would kick in---and the energy had to go somewhere in the body (especially since I would never run away from anything but just stand there, statue-like); it would manifest itself as severe pain in the muscles and joints.

Bullying

I'd already included several examples of me being bullied in school---by students and teachers. Bullying is quite common for a lot of kids, but for kids on The Spectrum, it's a bit more common and severe. Rarely, can we communicate what just happened much less try to talk our way out of a threatening situation. It's called a lack of self-advocacy in that we aren't able to stand up for ourselves. We need someone (a parent or brother or friend or...) to stand up for us or speak out on our behalf. This bit does improve over the years, thankfully. I can switch into a more aggressive mode, but it is a very slow, inclining switch as opposed to a kind of light switch with instant reaction. Nearly all of my bullying incidents happened in school.

There was a time when I was standing in the cafeteria lunch line, and an older kid told me to hand over my lunch money. I started to cry, and he felt so sorry for me, that he apologized and became a sort of protector of mine from time-to-time. That was unexpected. Another incident occurred at a day care. The one-and-only time my parents attempted to use a day care facility was a bit of a nightmare for all of us. I hated it. I did not and could not interact with the other kids there. I was mute. I stayed near the only thing I could relate to in the room: the TV set. Later that same night, one of the kids ran straight at me and tackled me to the floor for absolutely no reason (completely unprovoked) --- when I hit my head, I ended up with a minor concussion and had to go to the hospital. My parents pulled me out of the day care the next day.

Another incident was on the school bus in Middle School. This particular kid would torment me, daily, with name calling and occasionally throwing objects at me. He threatened to hit me, once. I was just quiet. I think that was the problem. My stillness and silence provoked something aggressive in this boy that I can never understand.

One day, as I was boarding the bus, the bus driver told me that the boy was in the emergency room---severely injured in, I believe it was an automobile accident with his family, but I'm not 100% certain of that. He was severely injured, that much I knew. The bus driver said: "you must be really happy about that." I answered her as matter-of-factly as I normally would have: "no. I'm not." I was raised to never rejoice in my enemy's transgressions. This was a rule I continue to stand by (that's not to say I don't enjoy the relief of an enemy's departure). I never saw that boy on the bus or at school since then.

I do believe most bullies in school eventually grow out of it---grow out of their aggressiveness---and often forget they were even bullies. Those of us who were bullied, however, NEVER forget it.

Religion

Here's a tricky subject. While growing up, I was essentially raised in a Pentecostal family. We weren't holy rollers or that hardcore about our faith, but we were devoted. We went to church every Sunday and talked about the other church members like everyone else did. I was taught to believe a certain way, and I simply accepted that way without question. It was the rule. I don't question rules. I didn't understand that there were social rules even in a place built to focus on a creator and not one another---but, that wasn't really the purpose, was it? This was another social interaction institution that had very specific start times, rituals, dress codes, speech patterns, and a host of other nuances that a kid like me could barely comprehend even when it was blatantly explained to me.

Once, I brought my glow in-the-dark Dracula toy to Church. I didn't realize it would be such a big deal and make such a negative impression on the fellow churchgoers. You'd have thought I brought a bazooka into the congregation. I kept my Dracula toy in my left hand and played with him while ignoring the boring sermon, standing only when we were expected to sing along to the hymnals (which I only read along to and never sang to). One couple even suggested that I never bring "an object of The Devil" into Church, again. My parents were upset by their reactions to a simple toy.

Over the years, I've collected various reasons to never step foot into another church. I found there to be a great deal of hypocrisy, backstabbing (not literal), lying, jealousy---essentially, all of the 9 Deadly Sins were found grouped into one building among people gathered to fight the very thing they unwittingly brought with them every Sunday and Wednesday.

I've embraced a CoS &Taoist philosophy and incorporated the simplistic, nature-based mindset into my beliefs and leave things as they may be. Apart from that role, I have little use for organized religion and consider it---of any kind---to be the root cause of many wars, forms of discrimination, and oppression. My intent is to not insult anyone else's belief. If he/she wishes to believe a certain way, so be it.

There was a situation where, during one of Dad's bible study classes he would conduct after-hours at a church, one of the members was telling me about a book she read. She said "it really makes you rethink how you look at things… makes you question what you've always believed." Me (not pause at all): "why would I want to?" Her reaction, I interpreted, was shock---she squirmed in her seat a little, looked down, and said "oh… well… that's a good point…" It never occurred to me that she was trying to be helpful; instead, I stated the obvious answer without concern over hurting her feelings.

Relationships

This base human need is essential for internal development, social growth, and longevity [3]. I've only recently had greater success with a relationship. I didn't start concerning myself with dating (although, attraction was there since I was 11 years-old) until I started high school. Suddenly, it was essential to be dating someone. It was perfectly fine to be alone or hang with friends prior to 9th Grade, but upon starting high school, it became a required social expectation. Anyone not dating someone was considered "a loser" or "a freak" among other colorful metaphors.

My world had already been rocked by transitioning from 8th Grade to 9th Grade as I was in a completely different environment that required new routines, new routes, attempting to memorize new faces, and changes in timing. All of the tricks and adaptations I learned were now meaningless. I had to start all over again.

"Normal" students didn't have this problem. They entered high school armed with a repertoire of communication skills, some sense of sexuality, and plenty of cross-reference experience. Those of us on The Spectrum do not have these tools to work with. All we have is adaptation or survival (flight or fight). We typically enter a new environment with a need to change it or retreat from it---there is no alternative.

I didn't have a sense of self-worth as far as physical appearance was concerned. I looked in the mirror, and I saw something quite unattractive and disproportioned. How accurate was that assessment? I believe I was far too critical of myself. How can one read himself when he can't read others? If a person struggles with social queues, body language, nuances, implications, and subtle emotions, then how can that person possibly develop a sense of self-worth? The answer is: he becomes introspective.

I never went to Prom. It was absolutely out of the question. It bothered me that I had no one to go with, but there was no way in hell I would ask someone. It was impossible for me to recognize when someone was flirting with me. How was I supposed to know who to ask and how to ask her? I didn't bring these challenges home to my parents. Again, once I came home, school didn't exist anymore (except for home work and studying).

Missed opportunities are an incidental collection for us on The Spectrum. We reflect and rehearse and play events, conversations, and preemptive possible conversations… over-and-over… trying to study the meanings, trying to comprehend what we may have done wrong or done right, and hoping we don't repeat the mistakes we made at that moment. This is another example of a compulsive/perseveration trait we share.

There was one girl who---I guess she liked me---commented on my appearance and started off with saying "…not that I'm flirting with you, but…" I took/take things literally, so I assumed what she told me was true; she was not flirting with me because she said so. Years later, I've played that scene over-and-over in my head, and it occurred to me that she may very well have been… flirting with me at the time. A missed opportunity.

Another girl, while already sitting on her school bus, looking outside the window, shouted down at me: "hey, what's up?" I didn't say anything because I still struggled with finding a suitable answer to "what's up?" I walked up to the window and just looked up. She was already looking around at other students by this point, but when she noticed I hadn't moved from my spot, she got mad and said "Jesus Christ! I just said what's up. That doesn't mean I want to talk all day!" I was embarrassed from that outburst and quickly left the scene and avoided her from that point-on. A missed opportunity.

Another girl was standing outside her classroom with another girl and was staring at me while I was walking by. She said, loudly, "he's kinda' hot." I heard it but kept walking---was she talking about me? There's no way she was talking about me. She shouted out, this time: "hey, you're hot!" I kept walking and never looked in her direction. What was I supposed to do? What was I supposed to say? How does one respond to that comment? Another missed opportunity.

While I was living in Phoenix, Arizona, I was sitting in a movie theater. The movie was already in progress. There were two girls sitting right behind me, and they were talking and clearly not paying attention to the movie. One of them asked me what time it was. I told her: "one theurty." That 'e' and 'u' is intentional because I was impersonating one of my favourite actors' accents. I don't know why I said it like I did, but I did. This intrigued the girl's friend and asked me where I was from… that I had an accent.

I told her where I was from and resumed watching the movie. I never once turned to look at either of them the entire time, so I never knew what they looked like. All I know is they were interrupting the movie. One of the girls finally said: "hey, do you want to meet us outside?" Me: "sure" without hesitation---instant response---I didn't even give myself time to think about it.

I continued watching the movie. I heard them both get up from their seats and leave. I finished watching the movie. Roughly an hour-and-a-half later, I came out of the theater, expecting them to be standing there like they asked. They were gone. Another missed opportunity.

Journal Items:

1990. Apartment complex – very attractive woman in pool turned towards me and said something… flirtatious, I think… to me. I didn't know how to answer, so I just stared back at her. Her facial expression changed (bothered, I think), and she waded back to the other end of the pool with the other people. Missed opportunity, I guess.

1990. Attractive female showing us the apartment we were going to rent at the time and pointed towards the pool down below and said something to the effect of "…and, there's the pool for you, you big stud!" with a grin on her face – I didn't know how to interpret what she meant by that at all – stayed silent and kept staring at the pool. She kept looking at me, expecting some kind of reaction.

I used to sit in the car in the parking lot, waiting for Mom or Dad to come out from the store, and I would watch the other teens walking in groups with each other, laughing, touching, and interacting. I would feel an overwhelming sense of bitterness because they had something I did not… something I could not. I was very sad and angry back then. I was angrier at myself for being "a robot." I actually hated myself because of it. I was also angry at anyone else who could do the things I couldn't. Simple, natural things. Twenty percent of Americans, or about 60 million people, suffer from loneliness that is severe enough to become their main source of unhappiness. Loneliness is not determined by the number of relationships we have, but rather by our perception of how socially or emotionally isolated we are. For example, we can be surrounded by family, friends, and colleagues but still feel disconnected and unwanted [3].

I was in my 20's when I finally went on my first date. A girl who was socially awkward but more assertive than me made sure to introduce herself and ask me out. Ask me out. Just a simple phrase like that didn't make sense to me back then.

Ask me out... outside? Out... where? Hollywood films tend to sensationalize autistic characters and especially over-dramatize taking things literally; however, there is a base truth to it. Simple, literal phrases like that can trip someone like me up and make things uncomfortable and outright weird for the other person(s) attempting to engage me in conversation---outside my special interests. I felt sorry for her. I knew it was going to be as much of a struggle for her as it already was for me.

She had an extremely difficult time trying to "read me." She was regularly frustrated because I couldn't understand what she meant by nearly everything she said to me. She took things personally and was mad at me, often. I will leave out the intimacy portions because this is not that kind of book, but I was incredibly robot-like, rigid, mechanical... there was no natural movement or instinct or expression...

I was so nervous about getting so physically close that I wasn't aware my hand was around her throat, and I was close to choking her... I was hyperfocused on my other actions at the moment and not paying attention to what my hand was doing! Our relationship lasted only 3 months. When she broke up with me, I was numb. I didn't feel sadness or anger or want to talk about it. I simply acknowledged it for what it was and moved-on.

I was going through some fairly extreme sad points during that time, and a failed attempt at a relationship long overdue (keep in mind, I started nearly everything later than most of my peers which includes dating) only added to that sadness. I attempted suicide, but I will expand on that bit in another chapter.

My second girlfriend came along 4 years after the 1st attempt. There was no one in-between… nothing… no flings, no flirts, no dating apps, no… nothing. I met her in my freshman year in college, and she was quite bold in personality. She invited me to a small party that she and her friends were having at an apartment complex. I was dreading going, but I forced myself to do so. There were about 5 people in the apartment with 1 of them playing pool. I later found out the 1 playing pool was her boyfriend. Ahem. Immediately, I questioned why she was asking me out (assuming this was an example of "asking out") with her boyfriend right there.

What made matters even more awkward was my car decided to not start that night, and it was he who helped make a simple repair and get my car started. The girl talked to me quite a bit in class (I had 1 class with her) and asked me on several dates. Each time, I felt… uneasy about it. I kept thinking about her boyfriend who she claimed she broke up with. For me? Not a good idea. Again, I knew she'd be dating "a robot." As was the case in the first relationship, I was incredibly rigid, mechanical, and robot-like with intimacy. The thought of someone being that close, touching… that was a sensory overload I could not handle, and I would lockup.

I still had an issue with her dropping her boyfriend for me and coupled with my own struggles, I simply stopped talking to her. There was no warning. I went silent. I didn't return her phone calls. Our relationship lasted 1 month.

My third relationship attempt was 3 years later. I was still in college at the time, but I had discovered something quite special, called the internet. I came across IRCs (Internet Relay Chatrooms) and a particularly intriguing one called SciFi/Fan. It was filled with people just like me! They were each socially awkward, geeks, and imperfect, but seeking some sense of a social network of sorts. Unlike previous social attempts, I could actually SEE the conversations take place on screen.

I could take my time reading and comprehending the meanings because I could scroll my screen back and re-read what someone typed. This was an invaluable tool. In fact, I credit IRC as having given me a sense of purpose that was greatly lacking. I learned how to develop an actual personality and sense of humour through IRC in a way I never could, otherwise. It was through IRC that I met my 3rd girlfriend.

It wasn't long before we were visiting each other, and, after several months, I did something I normally would have never done---I moved to another city to live with her. That was, by far, the gutsiest thing I had ever done in my life, and I was terrified. In fact, her cousin once asked me how I felt about moving to another state to be with her, and I replied: "I'm absolutely terrified." I was smiling when I said it, so my facial expression was out-of-context with the verbiage.

The same issues I experienced with the previous 2 relationships happened with this one, only it took a little longer because I could communicate with this one more freely---could joke with this one and discovered I had a more in-depth, silly sense of humour than I ever realized. It was unfortunate, but I was still a mannequin in this relationship---still a robot. Our relationship lasted 6 months.

A couple of years after that failed attempt, I tried to date again and even experience the notion of flings. None of them were successful. I needed someone who could accept me for what I was and how I was. In 2001 I found that relationship, and it has been 17 years strong, as of this writing. I'm fortunate because most of my peers on The Spectrum never experience a solid, long-term relationship.

Education

I decided to add some of my musings about my past employment and future prospects in this chapter because work, far more than skill, requires considerable social skills---and they can make you or break you. Entering the workforce was an extreme challenge for me because my silence and inability to comprehend the subtleties and politics and dynamics of an inconsistent environment were overwhelming, and I would lockup, speak only when I was forced to, and remained focused on the tasks-at-hand.

I eventually developed talents that I applied to my employment that grew into a strong desire to educate myself (I took sociology, psychology, and communication courses to improve what I was severely lacking in) and to focus on a career field (Information Technology).

Like any other form of social interaction, employment was quite the struggle for me in the beginning. I preferred jobs that required repetition and/or use of my mind in a research-like/problem-solving or visual descriptive manner. The entire journey through employment has had its significant highs and lows, but I've been able to discover and develop unique strengths I never knew I had through the experiences.

I started my very first job as an usher at an outdoor concert amphitheater in Phoenix, Arizona. This was my first work-related interaction with people, and it was not always successful. I was given orders to "check everyone's ticket" before allowing them to pass into the main auditorium (reserved seating) area. I followed those instructions, literally.

There were two reasons I did this: 1) that's what I was told, so I assumed there were no exceptions and 2) I couldn't remember anyone's face. I was yelled at by one of the patrons and told by him to "REMEMBER MY FACE!!!" I had another patron make a fist at me behind my back because I insisted on checking his ticket before letting him pass.

I had another patron tell my fellow usher standing next to me "yeah, I'm not going over to him" because he saw me looking up at another area of the amphitheater out of the corner of my eye---apparently, it gave the impression that I was angry. I loved working there for the music acts, but I dreaded going to there for the people interaction.

Keep in-mind that I was very young and inexperienced with this type of interaction, so I had no idea how I was coming across to others. I lasted 1 year before leaving on my own cognition. After that, a period of depression kicked-in, again, but I decided to start college to help curb that sadness. I attended one semester and was quite content doing so, but our family decided to move back home, again, and I had to stop college for a time.

My next job (first job back home, though) was at a movie theater, and I absolutely LOVED it. I worked as a ticket-taker, cashier, usher, and eventually was promoted to projectionist. Being a projectionist---still---is my all-time favourite job. I not only was able to watch and listen to movies, I was able to run them. I loved studying how the projectors and film spools/platters (very large metal dishes that hold the film while it's feeding through the projector) worked. I learned the nuances of these devices. I stayed there until the place shut down.

It was here that I met my 2nd lifelong friend, Brian. He was instrumental in cross-training in martial arts with me (Ving Tsun Gung Fu and Judo), and we would train together once-per-week on weekends. When the theater shut down, I was quite sad, and some of us transferred to another "sister" theater in town, but the employees were far from welcoming. They were clearly setting me up for failure (not sure why) – they would stay in the back room and force me to be the only one at the counter taking/handling customers; one of the males took money out of the register, looked at me while doing it---with two girls standing near him, grinning strangely. I don't know if they were trying to set me up for internal theft (blame me) or if they wanted to see if I would tell on them. I did not. I resigned that day but didn't say why. I later encountered my manager from the theater and told him the story.

I was a full-time student for 4 years afterward, but did have a very temporary (1 month), seasonal job working a pet store kiosk inside one of the malls in Albuquerque,

New Mexico. The customer interaction was not unpleasant as most people loved their pets and wanted to buy various items for them, so it was often a happy interaction.

One day, one of my co-workers inside the main store (the kiosk I worked at was just an extension of the store) started talking to me. She was a beautiful girl. I was reciprocating as pleasantly and formally as possible, but I must have come across as flirtatious… I guess? Her boyfriend was leaning against the wall, and I didn't realize he was giving me "dirty looks" the entire time until I looked his way.

As blind as I am at reading people's expressions, even I could discern that he was quite upset about me being so pleasant to his girlfriend. Another incident occurred at the kiosk when I chose to wear jeans that had far too many holes in them in places that were a bit inappropriate---I was asked by Security to get a change of clothes before they would let me back into the mall. It never occurred to me that my clothing was inappropriate.

Again, these are things we are completely oblivious of until someone points it out to us---then, we can learn from those mistakes. If no one says anything, we will never "see" things from their perspectives. I worked at a toy store in the receiving department for about 3 months just before leaving New Mexico and was fairly content being behind-the-scenes and doing a very repetitious job.

I worked for 6 months at a baby furniture store and actually enjoyed what I did. Most of my focus was on inventory and furniture assembly. I loved putting furniture together and was quite good at it, albeit slow. I discovered I had the knack for technical design at this job when I was asked to figure out why the inventory system on the computer wasn't working properly---I redesigned the system layout and fixed the minor bugs in it and added this to my responsibility list. Unfortunately, the job paid very little.

I worked for various distribution environments since then, organizing layouts, developing data matrixes, data analytics, reporting, tracking, technical documentation, compliance documentation, internal company web portals, interactive training environments, and numerous project management roles. I quickly realized I should focus on one discipline and aimed for Information Technology.

After earning my Bachelor's and Master's degrees, I continued pursuing management-level roles. At various times, I had direct reports/teams that reported to me. As difficult as social interaction is for me, you'd think I would have struggled managing teams, but that was a strength---I was often given compliments for being approachable, trusted, easy to communicate with, and even comments such as "you're the best boss I've ever worked for."

Unlike some folks on The Spectrum, organization skills come naturally to me because I apply an outline format principle to everything I do (folder and sub-folder technique)… I group things into categories and sub-categories… even physical objects.

Workplace politics, on the other hand, were my absolute weakest attribute. Specifically, I was BLIND to politicking in the workplace. I didn't see, much less understand, the internal struggles and posturing and manipulating that sometimes occurs. I was simply trying to help anyone who needed help. I didn't understand that, by focusing on one department, I was angering another---vice-versa. I was caught in the middle, at times, of turf wars I didn't even see. Unfortunately, this sometimes "pulled me apart" and would wear me down because I was trying to help too many people at one time.

My eventual solution was to automate each job I assumed---automated reporting, alerting, services, schedulers, etc. Once more, I was utilizing technical tools to aid my shortcomings. Another strength. On the flipside, because I have a very naïve viewpoint towards work ethics, I am invulnerable to manipulation---I keep it simple and get the job done.

Not being able to read body language and facial expressions or vocal tones (implied meanings behind them all) would be another huge obstacle. Interviews come into play, here, because maintaining eye contact, leaning forward, and having positive, confident body posture all contribute to successful interviews.

After conducting over 800 interviews in 1 year's time at a company I worked for, I realized I was far better at being the interviewer instead of the interviewee. As an interviewer, you have the control and advantage and little to prove. During interviews, as the interviewee, I would treat the sessions as simple question-and-answer scenarios where I would specifically answer each question but not elaborate without coaxing.

From my perspective, I already knew what I was capable of... already knew my strengths... but, it wasn't obvious to me that they did NOT, despite the fact I detailed my job experience in my resume's (often, at excessive lengths).

Taking things quite literally would get me into odd situations at times because I require very specific instructions if someone asks me for something or to go to a specific place at a certain time. If the person was too general, I had to fill in-the-gaps myself (and be right or wrong, 50-50, as a result) or continue asking for specifics until the other person grew impatient/angry with me.

At times, I would have difficulty interpreting the implied meaning someone would make during a conference call because I couldn't SEE what they were saying---as I point-out in later chapters, I need to see things in order to comprehend them; if they're spoken to me, it takes much longer for me to process, and if I'm not given the time to discern what I've heard, I may answer incorrectly.

I've since learned how to write things down every time I answer the phone or when someone comes into my office and tells me something---I instantly pull out a piece of paper and a pen and jot-down (bullet points) of what the person is saying.

The most consistent feedback I would receive from my bosses during quarterly and annual reviews was that I was too overwhelming in my communication. I would send very detailed emails that had images and video embedded in them to explain various processes or issues. I learned to cut that bit down into bullet points, instead, which was better received.

I avoided work-related parties. I used to come up with excuses or simply not show at the functions. I've since learned it's much more effective to simply state that I don't go to work-related parties. I don't explain why. The biggest thing for me is that everyone is taken out of context (out of work mode), and that throws me off, considerably.

A bad habit I used to have at work was simply entering an office or office area without announcing my presence. I never used to even acknowledge anyone was there but would go straight to the area I needed to work at, do what I intended to do, and simply leave.

The grandkids of one of my co-workers called me a "ninja" because I would slip into the room, work on the computer or router, quietly, and seemingly disappear without them knowing about it. Again, looking at things from others' perspectives is a never-ending chore because, from my own point-of-view, I was just accomplishing my objective as efficiently as possible.

At work, I've shocked many people (unintentionally) by just appearing behind them or somewhere out of their fields-of-view. They turn, jump or make some kind of surprised sound, and usually end up saying "oh, I didn't see you standing there." I've since learned how to knock on a door or a wall or a desk to announce my presence.

Going-forward, I've managed to attain a few technical certifications (including Ethical Hacking) and pursue a PhD in Information Technology. They used to say that autism prevented people like me from attaining higher education and achieving some level of success in employment---where it is a constant struggle, it is most certainly attainable.

In fact, it's in spite of that previous notion that I'm going as far as I can and refuse to hold myself back. I'm also taking the advice of a wonderful 104-year-old Polish woman named Mrs. Oppenheim, who told me to not stop at Bachelors or Masters but to get a PhD to set myself apart from everyone else---to give me as much of an advantage as possible.

Driving

I hate driving. It wasn't until I spoke to my neuropsychologist that I realized driving is, in fact, a social interaction. That explains a great deal. If you akin traffic to a crowd… someone cutting you off in a lane to someone being rude to you in a lunch line… having to understand the rules of the road to understanding the rules of social decorum… then you will see the similarity. It makes perfect sense because the same people are driving behind vehicles, and every nuance will transfer from them to their vehicles and their behaviour on the road.

Essentially, driving is a stressful endeavor for most people---for me, it's far stronger.

I enjoy driving certain cars, but I cannot stand certain things that occur on the road involving other drivers. In fact, weather conditions rarely bother me; I can deal with driving in bad weather. I cannot deal with the random, unpredictable nature of other drivers. Most of them drive with sheer impulse and impatience. Most speed wherever they go only to wind up at the same stop point as the rest of us. I do not believe the human brain is evolved enough, yet, to allow easily distracted drivers to effectively navigate from point-to-point without being involved in collisions or near-collisions. The thought of someone being distracted and looking in a different direction from the one they're heading---and swerving just a couple of feet toward another car---is enough to make anyone nervous.

For me, following the rules of the road make perfect sense. They're there for a reason. If they are broken, there will be consequences. In another chapter, I expand more on the importance of routine when it comes to driving---following the same routes to the few places I drive to/from.

There are very specific things that can trigger a slur of obscenities from my mouth:

Pulling up to a stop/intersection to turn onto another road while a large group of cars are arriving at the same time, forcing me to wait. This looks silly, but I notice it happens almost constantly/ consistently, and it enrages me. What are the chances of this happening as often as it does? Interrupting routine.

Drivers who don't use their turn signals when switching lanes. Not following rules/interrupting routine.

Drivers who ride my bumper in the left lane, and when I switch to the right, they pass me and pull into the right lane, anyway (they could have done that to begin with). Bullying/interrupting routine.

Drivers who wait until I'm approaching in my own lane---then, suddenly, pull out in front of me (they could have switched lanes a long time ago). Why wait until I get there to switch lanes? Interrupting routine.

Prosopagnosia

It (also known as 'face blindness') refers to a severe deficit in recognizing familiar people from their face [4]. This mouthful of a term is significant for those of us on The Spectrum. Not all of us suffer from prosopagnosia, but many of us do to varying degrees of severity.

Even though, during my neuropsychological diagnosis, I tested high with pattern recognition, I cannot recognize most faces, and this puts a tremendous damper on social interaction of any kind. The image, below, is only a slightly exaggerated rendition of what a crowd looks like to me.

At first glance, in particular, I can only see a sea of like faces that have little distinction. As I'm passing through a crowd, I don't make the effort to recognize anyone. I'm only interested in passing through… getting to my destination… then I slow down, rest, and take more time to study the faces in the crowd and maybe recognize a few.

I find that, after several minutes of scanning the same faces, over-and-over, I eventually do recognize some people and eventually recall past conversations with that person(s). It's actually quite terrible, this condition. Couple it with forgetting names, and you have a recipe for social awkwardness and failure.

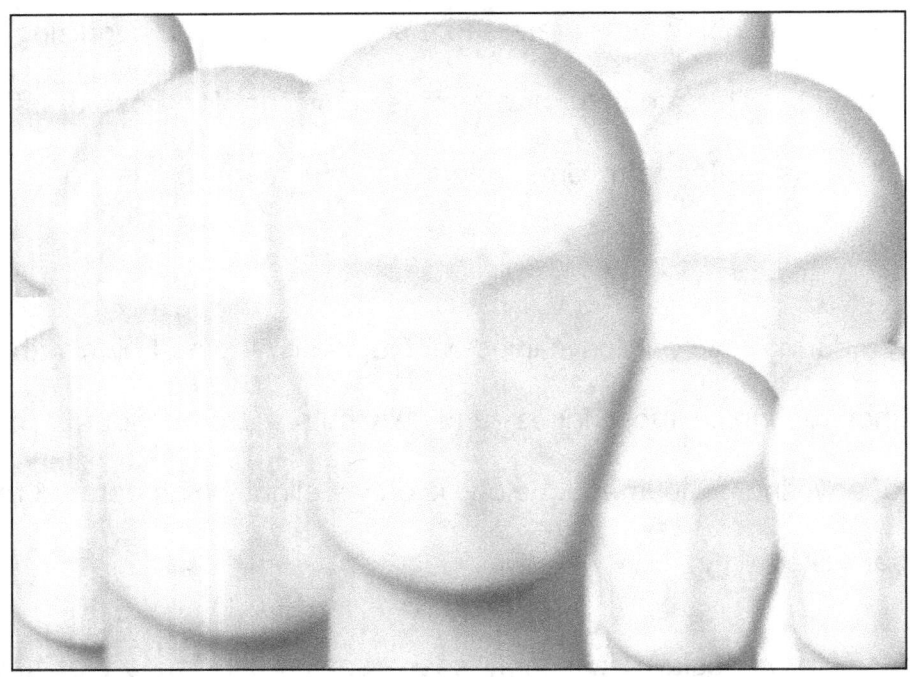

I can't guess age very well at all.. don't even bother to try. Can't recall faces but can recall voices. I've been able to recall meeting someone after they've spoken in combination with his/her face. I can't "see" myself in the mirror most times – not like others see me or cameras (especially) – I use three different mirrors in the house because, sometimes, it seems as though I look different in each one – believe it's the lighting differences in each room that are throwing me OFF – how I perceive myself sometimes conflicts with how I look in someone's camera photo (they may take of me with a group of others) – often, I think I'm smiling in the photos when I'm NOT – often my hair looks different than how I saw it just an hour/half-hour earlier at Home.

I've often confused one person for another---even people I've spoken to for some time (happened often during school because most of the kids looked alike to me).

I've asked a couple of friends on numerous occasions: "do we know them? I sort-of recognize his face…" They tend to get frustrated with me because I do it so often. I've grown to simply not ask at all and "roll with it."

I am fortunate that there are some people who have a separate diagnosis for Prosopagnosia and suffer far more severely from it. At least, over time, I can burn someone's face into my rote memory.

Journal Item:

2015. Former co-worker at ABSG at Costco approached me and knew who I was... I had NO recollection of his face... he changed his appearance slightly? I had to fake it... think he realized I didn't remember him

2015. Former co-worker at ABSG at Kroger came up to me with a big grin on her face... I vaguely recognized her... had to fake it for a couple of minutes while she fed me more info to cross-reference... looked at her name tag... Kelly... began remembering her... worked with her for couple of years

12/29/2016. After walking out move theater with two friends, a man walked up to us with a female and said "hey! It's a tattoo convention!" He asked 1 friend how his tattoos were then waved at me. I realized he was the tattoo artist who did mine in January. I couldn't recognize his face until it was in context. He spent 1.5 hrs. on my tattoo, and I couldn't even recognize him.

2016. Once I didn't even recognize ME in one of Sandy's photos at a pool party – I see this person I definitely didn't recognize at the party talking to a friend next to the pool – and realized it was ME in the photo. That was disturbing. I didn't recognize myself.

3/16/16. Coffee shop – been going there for years and recognize most of the staff – got two of the girls confused behind the counter – the first one told me she was stressed because she had to send an employee home and was understaffed – I told the other girl "good luck" thinking she was the first one – I replayed the event in my head after leaving the building and realized what I'd done…

2017. Lady approached me in line at the airport and said "hey!" She had a look on her face that I interpreted as one of recognition. I tilted my head and responded with my usual "hey" and kept looking at her. She paused for several seconds and finally said: "you don't remember me, do you?" She said her name, and it finally started to come back to me that she was the ex-girlfriend of a friend---whom I had dinner with on numerous occasions---I simply forgot what she looked like. Did she cut her hair? What was so different in just the span of 1 year that I forgot what she looked like?

3/28/2017. Restaurant .. couple.. wife.. "I've seen you dozens of times, and at Brad's party, but I've never been able to say hi, so.. HI." I had no recall of either of them.

Meltdowns

I also refer to these as "explosions" because they are sudden, intense eruptions of rage that simmer almost as quickly as they began. It typically happens to me when something I'm very much into at the moment is interrupted: there is 1) an intense agitation followed by 2) a loud shout then 3) silence. Most of the time, for years, I was unaware I was even doing this until more people would give me feedback. Once I was aware of what was setting me off, I learned how to stop doing it (or, at least, quell the intensity of it).

There was one point where I was so intent on playing with my action figures that my mom yelled upstairs for me to come down, and I didn't answer. I heard her, but I couldn't stop what I was doing. She finally yelled louder, and I thundered back at her at the top of my lungs: "WHAT?!!!" She was visibly upset (even I could see that). I actually apologized for hurting her feelings (I normally never apologized).

There were times when I would interpret someone raising his voice over the loud music I was listening to as actually yelling AT me, and I would be set-off, instantly, as a result.

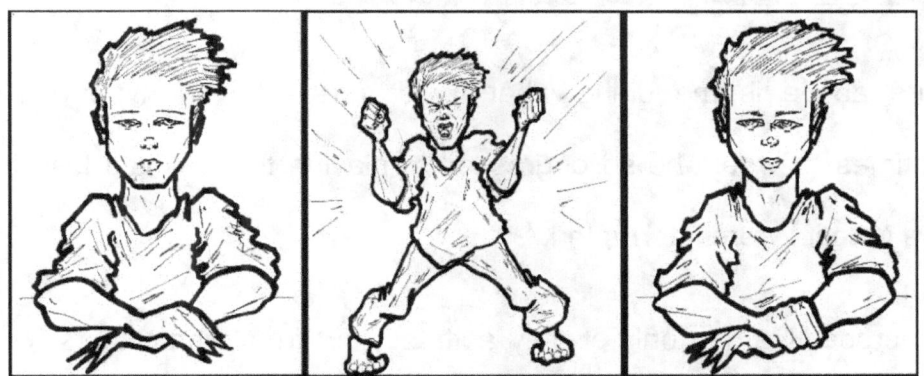

Meltdowns can also occur when I'm deeply frustrated with something. This goes well beyond a typical frustrated moment like most people experience. If there is something not working right---like it should---something that is no longer in sequence (which makes it instantly unpredictable), I lose it. It is far more intense than a temper tantrum. My entire body starts reacting (intense pain in the joints, coughing from a tightness in the abdomen, and sometimes sweating).

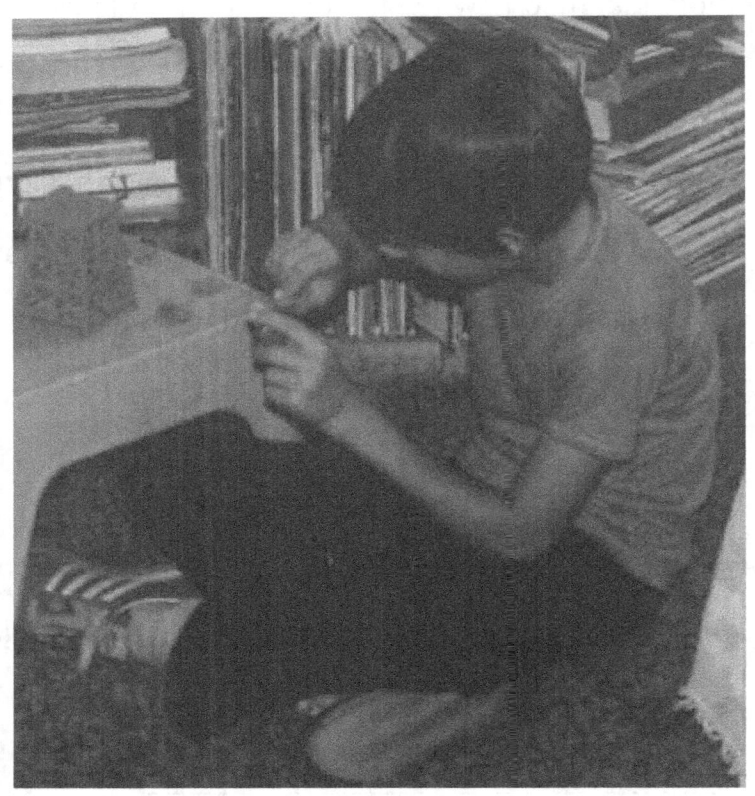

The picture above is me doing what I did most---remain hyperfocused on something at all times. I would be so engrossed in playing that I would lose track of time and get quite irate if I were interrupted.

From my perspective, I'm only slightly agitated, but from what others have told me, it looks like I'm in a flying rage. Thankfully, up until just 2 years ago, after learning what may have been causing these sudden interruptions, I learned how to stop them.

Social Gatherings

Contrary to popular opinion, most of us on The Spectrum actually do want to socialize, and we do try to socialize. For some, it's simply a matter of overcoming the awkwardness and restraining the over zealous speech or body space issues that accompany the attempted socialization. For others (I fall into this category), it's forcing oneself to endure something that you want to do but know full well will cause some form of anxiety while doing so. For me, there is a price to pay each-and-every single time I interact with others, physically and socially---which nearly always equates to fatigue, lockups, or muscle pain.

As a toddler through early adulthood, I would simply go mute each time or say as little as possible (one word, quick responses). As an adult, I still have the tendency to talk AT people through information exchange rather than TO people. I try to anticipate questions and premeditate my answers. If someone asks me a question, then it's quite easy for me to reply with something because Question-and-Answer is much easier to deal with (pull from what I've read or watched or heard); if someone makes a statement of some kind (even a compliment), that may throw me off for more than a second, and in the world of communication, that can cause an unusual reaction in the other person. If the person hits on one of my special interests, I slip into a sort-of encyclopedia mode and start rambling-on about that particular subject. If the person starts-off with an obvious statement (like the weather conditions), I will agree or disagree and leave it at that with little-to-no expansion on the topic to keep the conversation continuing.

Folks like me want to be invited and included, but once we go (party, club, concert, etc.), the endeavour becomes a sometimes-rewarding BATTLE. It's rewarding in that I am able to actually do it and complete it; it's a battle in that, especially if I've never been to the location AND recognize the people at the location, most of my time and energy is spent looking for that one perfect spot to stand near or sit at.

Greetings and goodbyes and small talk are simply silly practices to me. It's pointless to walk into a room and suddenly say "hello!" It's pointless to tell someone "goodbye" before leaving. I struggled with greetings my entire life. The natural reactions and verbiage "normal" folks employ require prep-work for someone like me--- and, if we'd never heard the word/phrase before, that's when the taking things literally stereotype tended to kick-into reality. The greetings "what's up!" and "sup?" puzzled me for the longest time. I wouldn't literally look up when they would say it, but I had no response. I would just stare back at them.

The very few times I experimented with saying hello to someone, first, instead of having to reciprocate (e.g. wait on them to start the greeting process) didn't work out well. The other person would either ignore me or not hear me (when I did attempt to speak my voice was high-pitched or low-pitched but barely audible). I would tell myself after each failed attempt that I would never do it again. To this day, I wait for the other person to initiate a conversation or to say hello.

The notion of small talk is absolutely baffling to me, and I'm only capable of it if--- if---the other person engages a special interest of mine. It seems completely pointless to discuss something that is commonly shared like the weather. Everyone experiences the weather at the same moment, so commenting about it makes no sense to me.

Other silly questions like "how are you?" are completely silly because most people are not really interested in knowing---really knowing---how well you are at that moment. The typical response: "fine. How are you?" is equally pointless. It's a hollow experience. Get to the point, please. I play this same silly game because I HAVE to, but I'd just assume we discuss direct matters and be done with it. This, too, touches upon empathy deficiency in that someone like me has little care for the other person expressing feelings during greetings or goodbyes.

An important item to include would be the numerous fun experiences I had with my parents. They were, after all, my best friends and not JUST parents. They were very young when they had me, and, in a way, we all grew up together. Some of my fondest memories were going to one particular nightclub in Albuquerque, New Mexico called Midnight Rodeo (shut down since then), and I absolutely LOVED the place.

There was no way I would've gone there by myself, so I would go with my parents. We would all play pool, dance, have some cocktails together, and enjoy the country music. I loved how dimly lit the place was and loved looking at the neon lights/signs they had throughout the place. When it shut down, a part of my good memories shut down with it.

Social interaction can be exhausting. Example: while attending a very large party---one of 3 days' worth of social interaction for the Kentucky Derby---I was among my small group of friends. I was already exhausted from the previous night's activities (having gone to one house party and a dance club), and I was absolutely overwhelmed the entire time. Apparently, it was noticeable by the commentary I was given by people I knew and people I did not know. I'd seen most of their faces for years, prior, so I recognized most of the folks there.

Others, apparently, I had met a few times before but could not recognize their faces. One person I had to associate with another just to recognize who he was and the fact I had spoken to him once before. Therein lies the very unfortunate effect of prosopagnosia, and it can be detrimental if the other person recognizes you (especially by name) when you can't reciprocate. Even worse, there is no way of explaining this to them.

Journal Items:

12/4/2016. Christmas party - I went with friends... . I knew several people... I "hugged" the walls... quiet... listening from conversation to conversation. I was usually standing behind/near one friend while he did the talking... one person tried to help me talk to someone new... simple basic questions... Me: I only answered the person's questions but couldn't converse further... Me: I didn't "open up" until after two drinks... I became a "social butterfly" afterward... initiated conversations but overwhelmed 2 people with topics about science fiction/ movies

12/7/2016. A planned get-together with friends... I barely said a word to anyone apart from rehearsed greetings... stayed at table when others came in... didn't say "hi" until they came to table... I had 3 Mosquito Margaritas... became more chatty... there were a few jokes/sarcastic statements made by the others that I could not understand

12/17/2016. Christmas party with known people... friends and familiar acquaintances... typical sensations. . scan everything and everyone... smile-

smile-smile... had 2 drinks... able to converse... sat at same chair at same table as last two years... One of the ladies also sitting at the table: "that's YOUR chair anyway... you always sit there.." Pictures taken... asked them if I was smiling... danced freely... Very comfortable with that group... mostly females..

12/26/2016. Christmas party - I recognized several faces... still quite/noticeably awkward... 3 cups of red wine helped... went on in depth long discussion with two people about 1940s vocalists... Jo Stafford esp... . history of the singers... Sinatra... Tommy Dorsey... They said: "you don't look old enough to even know about that music." I went into discussion about Art Garfunkel... (video of Disturbed singing Sound of Silence started it all)... Said some funny ad-hoc one liners... Wait for others to extend hands... Eye contact... must maintain.. Lights too bright upstairs... Others hugged me several times... . hate hugging... . patted twice on the back each time I hugged back..

12/29/2016. Tattoo artist said to me: "don't leave me hangin' man... don't leave me hangin'.." with his hand outstretched to me... Me: I paused... looked at his hand... . (oh... he wants to shake hands!) and shook his hand

1/23/2017. Cruise ship - awkward interactions – meeting new people – invited to several room parties and dinner parties on this vacation/cruise – part of me wanted to interact; part of me did not because I knew the outcome: 1) smile a lot even when not supposed to or 2) "frozen face" when not supposed to; 2) wait for someone to extend his/her hand – look down at hand – don't squeeze to hard or not hard enough; 3) forget name; 4) forget eye contact; 5) reciprocate voice level and excitement if possible; 6) answer all questions honestly but forget to ask questions in return/in-turn (even thought I may never encounter this person again). Had a very difficult time navigating the party crowd – tried to align my body so the traffic flow would not interrupt – sit in corner – too awkward looking – stand by door – too many people coming-and-going – listen-in on conversations near me – try to notice distinctions in faces, tattoos, hair, clothing, body types, smell of food, music – must look up a song I like – attempt stimming to calm down – being touched but not reacting – too focused – given compliments on various items (like necklace) but never said "thank you" because I didn't make it myself – explain how long I've had it instead or where I got it from. Someone sat on the couch next to me because I "looked lonely" and asked me several questions – I thanked him for taking the time to talk to me.

1/27/2017. Exhausted from the trip – exhausted each day after there was considerable public interaction (e.g. room parties we were invited to – dinner parties at guest tables – meeting new people at pool/hot tub) – no exhaustion when in routine – when not having to interact – no muscle pains either. Friends commented on how much I slept during this trip – I had to explain that all of the sights, sounds, and interactions were exhausting

3/22/2017. I couldn't read front desk lady's non-verbal queue that she wanted me to open the window… she had to tell me… I stared at her hand when she was motioning to the left repeatedly… I did not know what she wanted

5/4/2018. While at a house party – hugged by someone I've known for years – he noticed how stiff and distant my reciprocating hug was: "that was a HUG... we're on hugging terms... it wasn't inappropriate touching (he was laughing while saying this)." I guess my reciprocating hug was that of a kid afraid of being touched by someone else. Will I ever master the art of hugging?

5/5/2018. At another house party – finding the right wall to lean against – lineup against the walls – find a corner – too many people – too much touching – everyone happy and boisterous – too loud... way too loud – go outside where it's raining but there's air – can breathe better now – not noisy – want to go back in and "mingle" but can't – want to go home and go to sleep – not supposed to yet. Someone passed by and accidentally grabbed my arm and commented about how stiff it was (my arms and whole body were fully tensed-up every time I went back inside). Someone else said: "it's a party. You can smile." My response: "that's exactly why I'm NOT smiling."

5/6/2018. Absolutely exhausted but no muscle pains from the previous days' activities – staying home all day

There is a near-constant internal dialogue that nearly all autistic folks go through. We are constantly analyzing and over-analyzing our environment and the people in it. We are constantly guessing and second-guessing ourselves and others, and this internal dialogue contributes greatly to our slowed-down processing speed. It's a major contributor to our delayed responses at times.

Journal Item:

3/23/2017. Coffee shop... kids inside had strange looks on their faces... Staring at me while I walked in... one of the girls was taking a picture of me with her cellphone... they were whispering among themselves... after replaying it in my head... I concluded they were not making fun of me... I reminded them of someone.

Part of that internal dialogue involves accidental staring at other people. I do this on a regular basis. I can be thinking of something unrelated to what or who I'm looking at, and I suddenly realize I've been staring at a person the entire time. Once, when I was about 12, I freaked a lady out because I was locked on her face but replaying a conversation that happened near me, prior. She has an obviously-disturbed look on her face, turned quickly, and walked away.

In the following photo, you can see me in the middle of a large group of people (many were cropped-out from the sidelines). This was a 2018 Derby party that I was invited to due to association with other friends. I stayed by propped up by that beam for a long time, watching TV. In my mind, I was socializing because I was actually there with the other people… in my mind, I was socializing even though I hardly said a word. This is indicative of my entire life's experience regarding social interaction. Being… there… but not really there.

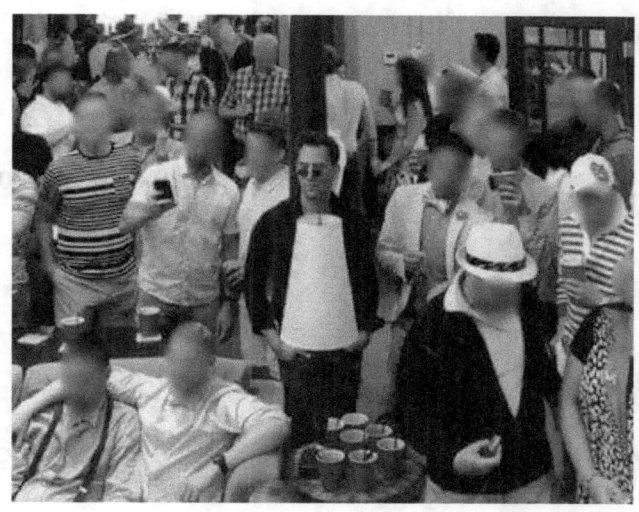

Dysphoria and Suicide

Here's a serious, touchy subject that most people are inclined to avoid. Deep down, they know that once a life has come to its end, that's it (at least, in the physical realm). I'm not going to get into spirituality (my beliefs have altered, considerably, since my old Pentecostal upbringing), so we're going to assume that once the body dies, it's dead… gone… and the impact is all that remains for those who are still alive. That's the power of suicide.

Depression can certainly lead to suicide, but it isn't always a direct contributor. Many people live with depression but have no intention of taking their own lives. They do suffer, however, and that can be a kind of living death all on its own. Unfortunately, depression (varying levels) is a part of being on The Spectrum. The cause can vary, too, because the frustrations of not quite fitting-in may be the biggest contributor.

For many of us on The Spectrum, we have a state of dysphoria (a low-level constant state of general dissatisfaction) in that we have a lower-level type of depression. Whereas, depression hits in spikes and valleys (highs and lows) and is often triggered by something specific and has a root cause (including chemical imbalance), those of us who are dysphoric have learned to settle with things as they are and don't expect much improvement, overall. This can lead to suicidal thoughts.

In 1993, I tried to take this innocent life. In 1998, I tried to take it, again.

It puts things into a different perspective when I look at photos of my younger self (I hated taking pictures… I hated it… hated seeing how I looked because what was in the mirror was not what I saw in the photograph---which one was the real me? I'll talk more about prosopagnosia at a later point). It's difficult to imagine taking the life of someone that sweet and naive.

Some people don't know what it takes to reach a self-ending point. They don't realize how dark and empty the air around you become. They don't realize the hollow feeling inside that, both, aches and yearns for release. I simply describe it as a darkness.

The incident in '93 was due to me believing I would never be able to change or improve. I didn't have a goal in life, no direction, and everything I tried to do on my own or with help from a few folks failed. I hated being lonely. I had my family, yes, but I was lonely. I failed my first attempt at a relationship. I was watching everyone around me live their lives---normal lives---mine was not. I concluded there was no point in continuing, so I bought several bottles of sleeping pills and pain killers and tried swallowing as many of the pills as I could. Luckily, they weren't high dosage, and when

I went to sleep that night, thinking I wouldn't wake up ever again, I did wake up. It was 4:00 A.M., and I awoke to a spasmic shaking sensation.

My entire body was shaking. My head was shaking. My eyes were shaking. The room was spinning. I acknowledged these effects and went back to sleep. To my surprise, I woke up, late that morning. When I stood up, I realized I wasn't shaking as bad, except my head was still twitching, slightly, and I was still a bit numb all over and a bit pale. My parents had no idea this took place. I didn't say a word about it until a few years later.

In 1995, I started college, and I found a sense of purpose. College---or the thought of having goals to achieve and something worth living for---saved my life, quite literally. There is no doubt I would have attempted suicide again, and I may have a couple of times, in-between. I don't really recall.

Unfortunately, in '98, I hit another low point and tried to kill myself, again. This time, it wasn't a matter of not having a sense of purpose while being lonely. This time, it was the fact that I was lonely---and my parents were separating, and the notion of my only sanctuary in life was disappearing. I concluded there was no point in continuing, so I tried slicing my wrists. I had heard that there was a right way to do it and a wrong way to do it. Even though I tried to do it the right way, apparently the broken window glass I used was too thick and not sharp enough.

The glass didn't go deep enough in my skin to pierce the arteries. I tried several times, but it only hurt. Now, I had something worse to be upset about---I couldn't even take my own life. That really bothered me because there was no escape at this point. I didn't tell my parents about the attempt until a few years later. Their reaction was quite indescribable---they were beyond upset.

I have a second thing in life that saved my life and cured my need for killing myself, and that was moving away from all of the negativity in my life and seeking a new one. I found a new city to live in. I started my Junior year in college, entered the workforce, and slowly gathered a small circle of friends. I had a solid, long-term relationship.

I had purpose. I had family. It actually can end on a happy note, after all. That's why I added this very personal section in this chapter. I want others to know that the darkness can go away. Life is short enough without our trying to speed things up… might as well finish the journey.

Chapter Conclusion

Thank you for sharing this journey with me. As I conclude this this chapter, I'm hoping I've been successful in detailing how socializing can be quite difficult for someone on The Spectrum. In the next chapters, I will detail why.

SENSORY OVERLOAD

What is Sensory Overload?

Most creatures on this planet possess senses of some kind that differ based on environment, DNA, species, injury, etc. Humans are no different. We're taught about our 5 senses early in school. We adapt to them during infancy. We gauge how well they function with medical tests (eye tests and whatnot) throughout our entire lives. Sometimes, corrections and compensations are needed for one or more senses to function "normally" through the use of prescription eye glasses or hearing aids.

Some humans are born with slightly exaggerated senses. This is a major contributor to the autism diagnosis. Most of us on The Spectrum have one or more senses that are either hyper-sensitive (accelerated) or hypo-sensitive (dulled) that cause minor to major difficulty in our lives at an early stage. Often, the overwhelming sensation of bright lights or the excruciatingly-loud sounds in a room are perfectly "normal" to everyone except for the autistic person experiencing them. We call this sensory overload.

Sensory Overload is defined as sensory overstimulation that occurs when sensory experiences from the environment are too great for an individual's nervous system to successfully process or make meaning from the sensory experience [5]. I prefer to include under-stimulation in this category as it can have equal-and-opposite effects, as well.

The DSM-V defines it as restricted, repetitive patterns of behaviour, interests, or activities, as manifested by at least two of the following, currently or by history [1]:

- Stereotyped or repetitive motor movements, use of objects, or speech

- Insistence on sameness, inflexible adherence to routines, or ritualized patterns of verbal or nonverbal behaviour

- Highly restricted, fixated interests that are abnormal in intensity or focus

- Hyper- or hypo-reactivity to sensory input or unusual interest in sensory aspects of the environment

It is immensely difficult to describe to "normal" folks exactly what it's like to experience issues with the senses beyond the typical, infrequent agitation that all people experience. I have yet to encounter someone who prefers coarse t-shirt tags rubbing against the back of his/her neck. I have yet to encounter someone who enjoys standing outside in a rainstorm for a lengthy period of time. Most people don't respond well to having sunlight reflections directly in their eyes or the smell of days-old garbage outside their bedroom window.

For those of us on The Spectrum, very specific things not only agitate but can debilitate us. Picture any annoying sensation tuned-up to the 10th degree, and you now have some idea as to what we experience on a constant basis. One person in a forum described it as: "dodging paintballs all day." Another person described it as: "constantly walking through a minefield."

Imagine hearing the scraping sound of an indoor plant's leaves against a wall every time the bedroom fan blows against them---and having that wake you up from a deep sleep because it sounds like someone scraping a shovel against a brick wall. Imagine feeling as though someone is shining a spotlight directly in your eyes at close range every time the sunlight reflects against a glass sitting on a desk on the other side of your kitchen. Imagine the texture of sweet potatoes feeling more like wet mud against your tongue every time you're forced to eat the damned things. Yes. These were my own experiences. Many of us on The Spectrum are forced to relate, but I'm not trying to appeal to them; I'm trying to show everyone else what it's like.

Why? Well, perhaps a teacher or boss or parent or friend will better understand why certain people freak-out during very specific situations, seemingly for no reason. Perhaps, that one person will better understand why her child "explodes" in a rage whenever pudding brushes against his lower lip.

My parents had a bit of a workload whenever taking me to a movie theater or outdoor drive-in. They had to surprise me about it because I would get so excited (good and bad) about going to the show that I would typically throw-up. It happened numerous times. Surprising me about going didn't work too well because I would just throw-up while I was at the theater (or in the car while pulling up to the parking lot). I LOVED movies, but I guess everything tied to the environment was overwhelming. I never felt a sense of noticeable dread about going to these places, but something was causing the preemptive reaction. Was it the smell of the food at the concession stand? Was it the bright lights in the lobby? Was it the numerous sounds and music? It wasn't until I was about 14 years-old that I made a mental decision to stop doing that---to stop getting so worked-up---stop throwing-up! I can laugh about it, now, but that was quite a monumental effort of willpower for a kid to undertake on his own. My poor parents had NO idea what was causing it apart from me just getting so excited about going to the show (I'm actually laughing out loud while typing this, by the way).

Touch

I am extremely hyper-sensitive when it comes to touch---to anything brushing against my skin---especially things like the wind or the breeze from fans and air conditioners. I particularly despised the sensation of water against my skin when I was a child---so much that I refused to take showers and baths. I would simply avoid bathing for as long as I could until I had to sponge bathe and wash my hair at the kitchen sink (I would stand with my hands under the water for up to 15 minutes before putting my head under the faucet). Getting ready, as a result, would take up to 2 hours (nowadays, I can get it done in 1 hour).

I didn't really mind being held or picked-up as a toddler by my parents or grandparents. If anyone else came near me, however, I would simply lockup. By lockup, I mean that I would go incredibly stiff and numb. Just after I was born, our family doctor commented on several odd things about me: 1) I didn't cry 2) I gave him "looks that could kill" after he made me cry and 3) I was "stiff as a board" every time he or the nurses would try to pick me up. It's quite humorous to me that this trait never improved over time. I am still the same way.

I had a fascination with specific things and would do what I could to touch them. Anything hanging on walls or shelves, I would have to reach out and touch. Wall paintings were always crooked in the house, as a result. I took advantage of the height elevation I would gain every time Mom would pick me up and carry me through a grocery store, for example, as it gave me the distinct ability to reach out and touch the canned items on the upper shelves---consequentially, many items would be on the floor (sometimes dented) every time she would carry me down an aisle. She had to walk down the center of the aisles so that I couldn't reach anything.

Stockings were a curiosity to me. Many times, Mom and I would be standing in line at a store, and my hand would be gliding up-and-down the legs of any lady near me---if she were wearing stockings---because my little mind couldn't comprehend why certain people's leg colors didn't match the rest of their bodies (e.g. brown or dark or white stockings). The texture puzzled me. Needless to say, Mom had to explain my behaviour and halt it quickly.

As a kid, I hated toys that had material (clothing) of any type on them and would immediately take the material off. The plastic was perfectly fine to touch, but I couldn't stand holding an action figure (for example) that had clothing on. I hated the way it felt. I have no explanation why apart from it being a texture issue. My parents would come into the living room where I always played (same spot by the couch – I rarely ventured anywhere away from that same spot) and would find all of my toys completely stripped of their clothes. They thought it was odd and would comment on it, but it was dismissed as, yet, another oddity from me.

As a toddler, my hair became an extreme agitation. I didn't understand then why, when I would go outside, the sensation of my hair being blown in the wind would drive me absolutely bonkers. I would feel the hair strands moving against my skull (picturing an army of bugs crawling through it) and start gouging at my head, furious. It would be so bad some days that I would even pull some of my hair out. It didn't occur to me that it was the wind causing my grief until I reached about 12 years-old. I did know that fans, heaters, and air conditioners were torturing me each time they'd blow on me even at an early age, however.

During my teens, I discovered hair spray. That was a wonderful compensator in that I would use copious amounts of it to keep my hair from moving. One girl I knew called my hair "the helmet." If so much as a strand would come loose, I would freak-out and go out of my way to get even a small bottle of hairspray as soon as I could to spray it back down (water just wasn't long-lasting enough).

Driving. To this very day, it's common to find the vents on my driver's side closed and the passenger's side open. This is my solution for keeping the air from blowing on me while still keeping it circulating.

During childhood, certain fabrics would drive me crazy.

I despised collared shirts of any kind. I was forced to wear them, depending on what I had available to wear to school that particular morning, and I would spend my whole day tugging at the collar, trying to keep it away from both sides of my neck and throat (especially). It was not unlike having a tight hangman's noose around my throat. Ties were completely out of the question. Even to this very day, I wear shirts with collars quite loose and as unbuttoned as attire-appropriate as possible. I've had people describe the way I wear my ties as looking more like scarves because they hang quite loose/low away from my throat. Below, is a typical shirt of mine (that didn't have embedded tags) with the tags cut or torn out.

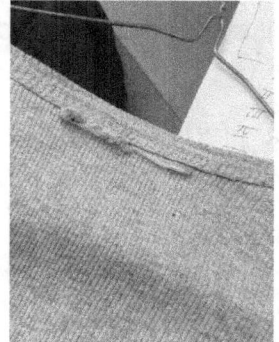

Back then, most t-shirts had coarse tags along the inner collar. I would rip them out as often as I could, sometimes damaging the shirt (because the tag would be stitched too deep into the shirt material) by tearing a slit all the way through. Me being the way I was, I didn't notice much less care that I had visible tears along my shirt collars. It would take days before my parents would notice, and it took a bit longer for them to realize WHY this was happening to my shirts (they caught me ripping a tag from a shirt right after buying it for me and told me not to do that again). I also avoid turtlenecks for obvious reasons but did force myself to wear them for a few weeks in the 1990s before throwing them all away (you can't say I don't at least try to fight this thing from time-to-time). Later, clothing designers started coming out with v-neck t-shirts and/or embedded labels. I never bought a single ring t-shirt since. V-neck t-shirts saved me a great deal of grief.

Other clothing items would drive me crazy, like mittens. I tried wearing them for one day, and I never wore them since. I couldn't stand having my fingers pressed so close together in a cramped space like that. I couldn't stand not being able to touch anything with my fingertips. To this very day, I only wear fingerless gloves regardless of the temperature or wintery conditions outside. I'll deal with the ice burns. Surprisingly, socks or boots don't bother me nearly as much. What isn't surprising is the fact that hyper-sensitivity is not across the entire body but is in specific areas of the body.

Sometimes, interesting side-effects come from uncomfortable origins. Because of my over-sensitivity near my throat, I learned to have very quick preventive reflexes when I was training in JiuJitsu. The moment I felt my opponent trying to slide his hand towards my neck, I would intercept his wrist and pop my head away.

Wallets and things in my pockets. It's incredibly rare that I will put something in my pockets. I carried a wallet for a very short while in my teens because I didn't know where else to put my ID and cash/cards. I quickly discovered "fanny" packs and was far more content strapping them around my waist and carrying everything in them instead. The sensation of a wallet pressed into me or keys in a front pocket or a wad of cash or paper... anything that took up solid space was immensely uncomfortable and just as aggravating as wearing jewelry. To this very day, if I put something in my pockets, it doesn't remain there longer than 1 minute before I transfer it to some other location (jacket inside pockets work just fine in winter). Since the invention of mobile cellphones and phone cases, I now use them to carry my ID/cards (in a plastic case that rests behind the phone) by clipping the case on my top pocket or waistline. I don't even wear belts (too restrictive).

Milk cartons. When I was a child, I couldn't open milk cartons because I couldn't stand the sensation of the carton---the material (just thinking about it right now gives me the shivers). I would start to pry the carton open, and if it opened without me having to touch the center portion, I was fine; if it didn't open properly, I would attempt to pull it open with my thumbnail, feel the horrific material against my nail, and drop the carton on the table or floor or whatever.... sometimes, I would even YELP at the sensation. At home, I had my parents or grandma to assist me, but at school I didn't have such a luxury and would sometimes ignore drinking anything during lunch just to avoid the sensation or use a pencil to poke a hole in the carton mouth and pry it open that way.

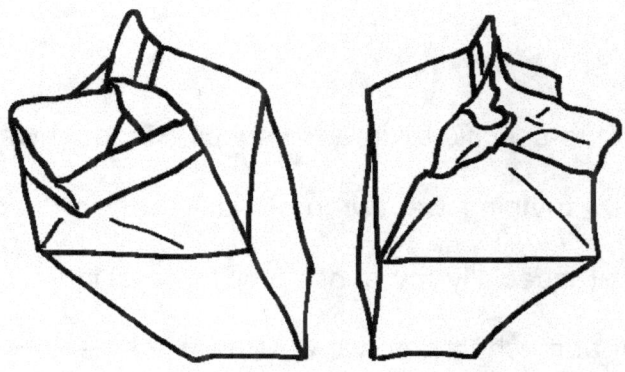

Oddly enough, nothing about the carton touching my lips bothered me.

Chalk. The touching, holding sensation of chalk. I despised holding chalk in my hands. I was rarely called upon in class, so I didn't have to hold chalk often through school, but when I did, I would have to focus on what I was writing on the board instead of the horrific sensation. I suppose a way of describing what it felt like (to me) is comparing it to.... well.... I simply cannot describe it. It wasn't painful; it was simply unpleasant as hell. The dry, flakey feeling and the fact it wouldn't come off unless washed off encouraged me to avoiding chalk whenever possible.

Speaking of texture, most folks don't realize that it isn't TASTE that freaks-out kids on The Spectrum---it's touch. The texture of certain foods touching the tongue is what usually triggers an unpleasant reaction. If the child is forced to endure it (e.g., forced to eat that food) a meltdown will more than likely occur. In my case, I refused to eat certain foods: raisins, tomatoes, and coconut---all due to texture. What is a meltdown? A meltdown is 'an intense response to overwhelming situations. It happens when someone becomes completely overwhelmed by their current situation and temporarily loses behavioural control [6].

Because of my hyper-sensitivity to specific textures in specific foods, I was quite underweight. My parents didn't think anything was wrong… just the fact that I was skinny. Most people would comment (especially my aunt): "you're so skinny!" I didn't really want to eat/didn't enjoy eating that much. There were some foods I enjoyed, but I couldn't keep eating them indefinitely (though, I would have eaten the same things, over-and-over, if given the freedom to do so); I was an average of 30 LBS under my peers' average weight.

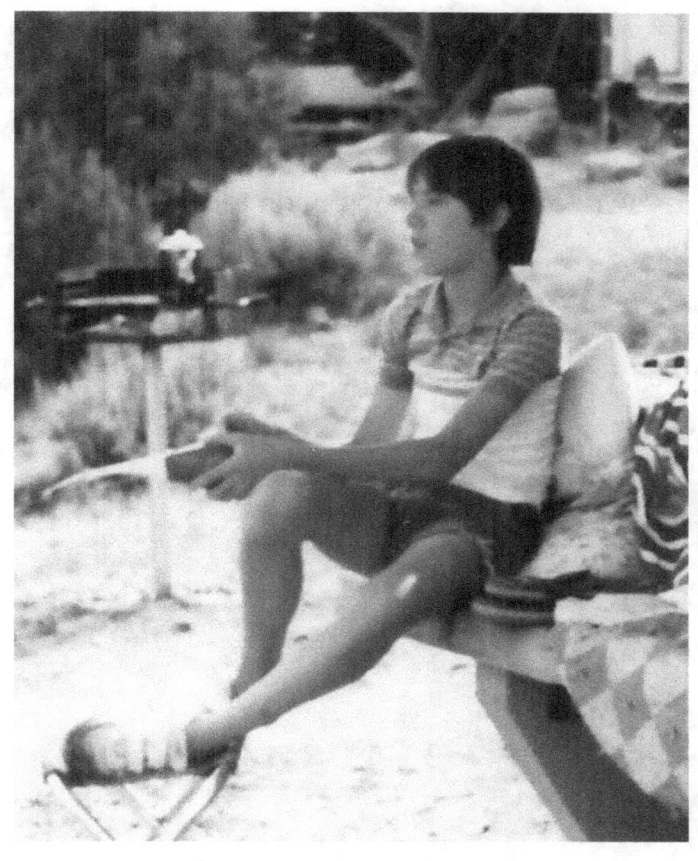

In 2nd Grade, I had a somewhat physically abusive teacher who saw my defiance for eating sweet potatoes as, well, an act of defiance. She didn't understand---how could she? I was incapable of explaining why I couldn't eat them. I couldn't explain to her that sweet potatoes felt like wet clay in my mouth. She yelled at me in front of the entire lunch room of kids to eat my sweet potatoes. I didn't say anything. I simply froze and stared at them. I wasn't embarrassed or scared; I was numb. She came up behind me, picked me up by the shoulders and slammed me down, hard, on the bench we were all seated at and told me to eat them one more time, standing over me at this point. I took maybe two or three bites and PUKED all over the tray and table. The funny part to this story (despite the negative context) is that my puking caused a chain reaction with the kids next to and across from me---each kid started puking on the table!

The teacher never forced me to eat anything from that day forward (she comes up in the previous volume, by the way).

As an adult, I can say I can tolerate sweet potatoes and tomatoes. Some things do improve over time.

As a kid, there were a specific style of jeans that I absolutely despised. They felt... weird to me. The hips were jutted-out as opposed to other jeans I wore, so I would only wear them when I was forced to. I referred to them as "Nazi jeans" because they looked like Nazi uniform pants (to me).

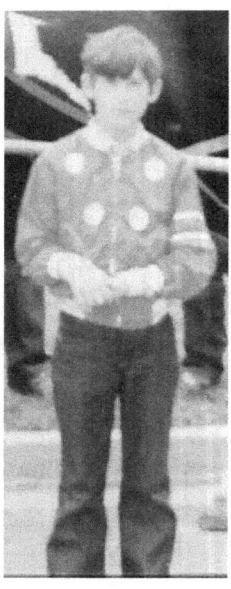

The photo above is one taken of those very same jeans. I'm leaving the brand name out on purpose. As you can see, they do jut-out at the hips to the sides. I envisioned them as two triangles at my hips. I didn't mind the flared legs below my knees---it was the hips I had an issue with.

Every step I took felt... weird. I can't put a better description to it, but the moment we gave those jeans away, I was ecstatic about it.

The dentist. There is a title that strikes fear in most kids' hearts, regardless of mental state. My parents attempted to take me to the dentist---once. That was a huge mistake. I completely freaked-out. My parents had to haul me out of the office as quickly as possible. I refused to go back---and didn't until 2003. The only reason I went in at that time was due to an abscess tooth. It was during that dental visit I learned how to apply my "stiffen up" coping mechanism while having all of those foreign objects prodding and digging inside my overly-sensitive mouth. My dentist even suggested for me to "go to your happy place." I've held onto that phrase ever since. To this day, I dread going to the dentist, but I keep up with my scheduled maintenance appointments. I do feel sorry for their chair arms because I crush them every time. The process I despise most, however, is the rinsing---I cannot stand having the suction tube in my mouth and closing it around that damned thing.

Journal Item:

1/19/2017 - dentist – HATE when they touch my hair while they're cleaning my teeth! Hate leaning back in dental chair – will flatten hair – very stiff rigid squeezing arm chair rests – not gripping chair hands contorted weird - stiff

Speaking of the dentist, I'd recently started wearing clear braces ("invisible" braces) because I do have a few crooked teeth that I wanted finally straightened. I did OK wearing them for the first 6 months. Something simply... halted me in my progress, however. It wasn't gradual. It was sudden. I simply could no longer wear the braces. I spent $3,000.00 on those things, and I'd wasted $1,500.00 worth as I stopped halfway. Having them in my mouth was just like having a boxing mouthpiece in. The sensation was overwhelmingly torturous. I would pull them out most nights. It was painful when it shouldn't have been and non-painful when it should have been. Absolutely aggravating. The only thing that kept me fighting-on was the before-and-during progress I'd noticed because they were actually working.

There was a very unpleasant experience with a doctor at a downtown medical center when I was about 5 years-old. I had a very painful earache, and the doctor was trying to examine my ear, and I would have none of it---I began screaming and resisting. The doctor got a bit rough trying to restrain me so that she could properly examine me, but I would only scream louder. The thought of someone touching my ear, much less restraining me, was more than I could bare, and I had a meltdown as a result. Mom had to pick me up and carry me out of the facility (she was angry at the doctor for treating me so rough, but I think if I had not reacted like I did, it wouldn't have looked so bad).

/Earbuds and earplugs. I still cannot put those damned things in my ears. It's like trying to shove metal cans inside my ears, instead. When you're hyper-sensitive (especially to touch), very specific things create very specific reactions, and they're unpredictable until they actually happen. It's no wonder I used to get so many earaches when I was a kid because I hated wearing anything over my ears (even earmuffs). Thankfully, these days, I've improved somewhat in this area and can, at least, wear slouchy beanies (they don't really bother me even though they are pressing against my hair).

Jewelry. I hardly wear it. I gravitate only to silver (because they don't really make black jewelry, per se') when I do wear it. I can't wear anything around my wrists or on my fingers---which pretty much eliminates bracelets and rings. Regardless of how loose they are, after about 5 minutes, I'll start feeling pain and extreme discomfort and will tear them off as quickly as possible. I can, however, wear necklaces as long as they're loose. I've been wearing the same Ankh necklace since 1989.

My mother used to cut my hair, and that was quite an ordeal for both of us. What should have been a 30-minute task would take at least 1 hour. I couldn't hold still long enough for an even cut, even though I was never hyperactive---I was nervous---I hated the sensation of the cold metal against my skin… the drops of hair against my neck or my eyelids. Eventually, she would just give me the "bowl" cut and be done with it. I didn't care what it looked like. I just wanted it done. RARELY, did anyone else cut my hair. There was a period where my parents took me to a commercial hair stylist, and I would be stiff as a board through the entire process. Having someone else touch my hair, forehead, ears, the back of my neck was absolutely agonizing. I completely stopped allowing others to cut my hair since 2003. I learned how to cut and style it on my own (vent brush, handheld mirror, blow dryer, mechanical clippers, and hair spray) and am quite content with this workaround.

I like to dance, surprisingly. It took me years to overcome the mental block that kept me from attempting it---the thought of expressing myself in a physical manner was unthinkable. Mom and Dad taught me that it was perfectly normal to dance. Expressing myself to music and vocals was challenging until I learned the beat and how to move to each beat. I learned to incorporate Gung Fu movements while dancing, and that helped a great deal. The primary thing that I struggle with, however, is having random bodies brushing against mine---even briefly. If someone just barely touches me while passing behind me through a crowd (not just on a dance floor), it's like a hundred alarms go off inside of me. I never emote when this occurs. I never retract like some people might. I do the opposite and lockup/go stiff, even briefly.

Speaking of being touched…

Even though my parents hugged me on a regular basis (affectionate family), I never really sought it out from anyone. I could go on through my entire life without ever having the need to touch another human being. This looks sad to read, I suppose, since "normal" people are tactile by nature. I watch others interact in conversation, and there is a surprising amount of touching that occurs---an occasional tap on a shoulder or knee or hand shake or… these things are quite puzzling to someone on The Spectrum. Why? When you're born with tuned-down frontal lobe genes (a common difference between autistic brains and "normal" brains) you grow up missing the elements that others take for granted. For us, we have to imitate whenever possible and manually tell ourselves to respond a certain way in certain situations, to manage our body language a certain way in order to look "normal," to say certain things so as to not insult others, and so-on.

Journal Items:

12/20/2016 - friend commented that I don't like to be touched… not comfortable with it… confirmed that I pat people on the back when hugging and keep a distance

Me: "how did you know that?"

Friend: "you keep distant when people get close to you."

1/16/2016 - (restaurant) sensory overload – crowded people walking back-and-forth a lot brushing up against me – have to keep moving out of way – found corner to stand at – tapping my fingers against each other (stimming) – focus on TV in corner – can finally breathe after being seated at table

Shaking hands. Words cannot describe how challenging this simple gesture is to someone on The Spectrum. Why do we so often not hear a person's name when spoken during a handshake? The answer is that we spend more focus on standing properly, reciprocating the extended hand, not squeezing too hard/not hard enough, remembering to make eye contact (because that's just what you're supposed to do in The States), that we do not hear anything spoken to us---we just hear "wa wa WAH wa." The repeat the person's name twice trick does work for some of us, but it certainly doesn't work for me. Although, this example falls in with the Social Awkward category, there is a physical involvement that is the root cause behind this particular constraint. We can practice this over-and-over, but the moment there is physical contact, all of the brain signals and nerves are firing-off in defense mode, overriding the multitask capability of the brain, restricting the other senses. In other words, flight or fight mode kicks-in, and there is no reasoning with survival instinct once that occurs.

Journal Item:

1/2018 - on the cruise a male caressed my hand (I think) instead of shaking it like most guys do – I stared at his hand while he shook two others, and he shook theirs differently

Greetings and goodbyes are simply silly practices to me. The notion of having to extend hands and shake, the measure of a grip is some kind of message to one another (hence: "wow. Good grip you have there!") and makes no sense---it never has. You're expected to maintain your gaze into the other person's eyes but not too long and not too short (too long is uncomfortable to the other person; too short is disrespectful to the other person). It's no wonder people like me fail this act far more often than we pass it. It's no wonder I forget the other person's name when I'm having to manually remind myself of these steps each-and-every time.

I've been in Martial Arts (special interest) since 1988. I'm perfectly fine interacting with training partners at a distance (long range, kicking; medium range, striking), but in the close range (trapping/grappling), there is a constant touch. I've calculated that it takes 15 minutes of touch before anxiety kicks-in, and I experience shortness of breath, intense sweating, muscle tightening and muscle fatigue. I simply dismissed it, for years, to not having good endurance---until I started researching and capturing the data. I soon realized it was all tied back to hyper-sensitivity and anxiety.

For me, any physical act requires aforethought. Intimacy is a challenge whereas I have to tell myself to extend my hand a certain way or to express affection or… it's all quite mechanical and not natural. Unless a significant other understands these challenges ahead-of-time, he/she is unable to deal with it and will undoubtedly assume it's his/her fault or get angry at the poor "robot" who's trying like hell to adapt as best as possible. My coping mechanism for being touched is to numb myself. I don't do this consciously. It's a reaction---flight or fight---in the brain that tells my body that I'm under attack. I go very stiff/rigid.

My walk is noticeably rigid and robot-like. Apparently, when I run, I look quite odd because I'm so stiff. In school, several kids called me "rabbit" because I ran like one. Once, a co-worker told me: "don't ever let anyone see you run."

Journal Item:

2017 - fellow gym member – called out behind me "sir. Sir." I didn't react because… I rarely react to random callouts like that I guess because I assume it's not me they're speaking to. In this case, it was. He asked me "what do you do for a living? You have a very confident walk." I told him I was just a boring IT Director. I'm assuming he thought I was in law enforcement or something that imbued me with a sense of self-confidence. The point being he noticed I walk differently than most other folks.

Some things improve over the years for us. Some things simply change but rarely go away.

I finally learned how to dial-down my rigidity while in public places after catching (and documenting) how hard I leaned on counters while placing an order (for example). One day, I looked down and noticed how off-colored my fingers were because I was pressing into a counter instead of just leaning on it---full force---like an isometric exercise. That's how stiff I would get just being in a public place---that's the power of anxiety. I learned how to recognize when I was squeezing my hands together behind my back too tightly (was told about this while I was addressing a room full of employees at work, once: "your hands were turning yellow!") and let-up on the pressure.

At Work, I would refuse to ride on the golf carts inside our shipping facilities because I couldn't stand the sensation of the breeze against my face, back of neck, arms and hair, especially. I would walk everywhere even when I didn't have to. When I ride in a vehicle with someone else, I'll insist they don't roll down my window (no matter how hot it is) so that the breeze doesn't blow against me. When I had longer hair, I would drive leaning forward with the seat leaning back so that it wouldn't touch my hair. There was a carload of people in a lane next to me who noticed how forward I was leaning in my car, one day, and I noticed they were all laughing at what they were seeing---that was my cue to maybe start leaning back a bit more. When people touch me, I "lock up" and get real stiff like a robot. When people hug, my response is very automaton-like with three "pats" on the back and a distant body space followed by a quick pull away.

Journal Items:

12/26/17 - others hugged me several times… hate hugging… patted them twice on the back each time I hugged back

1/1/2017 - they like to hug… I consciously reduced the back-patting… sat in corner near the group… introduced to a female… forgot her name the moment she extended her hand to shake.

Below, is an example of something I finally did in my office (work). I couldn't stand the sensation of the breeze from the air coming through the ceiling vent, so I stuffed each opening with foam. That was the best thing I could have done (apart from asking our Facilities folks to completely remove the vent).

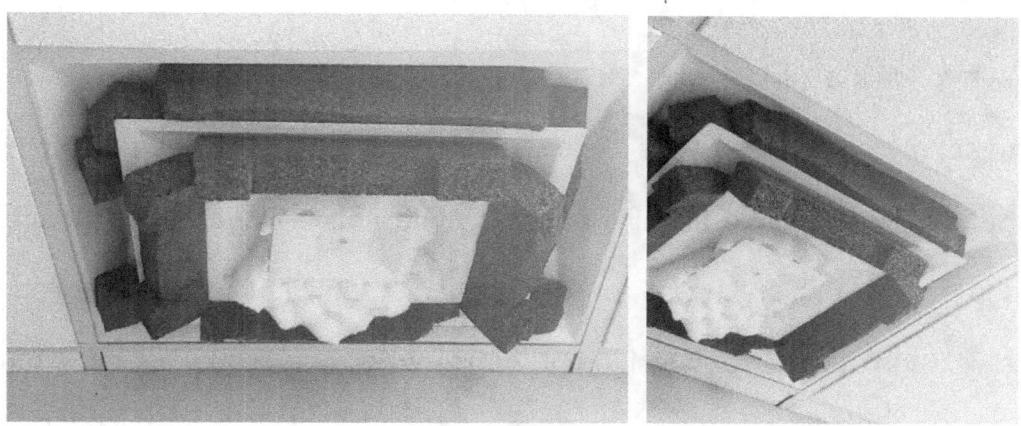

Wind. The wind is truly my nemesis. I don't think there is anything in life that brings me more torment. I spend a great deal of my time avoiding the wind, but it's rarely possible. I read weather reports, and if the wind projection is anything near 10 MPH, I put extra coats of hairspray on so that I won't feel the effects of the blowing nearly as much (ref. the section above regarding hairspray). If the wind projection is 19 MPH or higher, I'll do anything to keep from going outdoors. I've avoided social engagements, rebooked appointments, canceled going to the gym, gone through the drive-thru instead of going inside---just to avoid the wind.

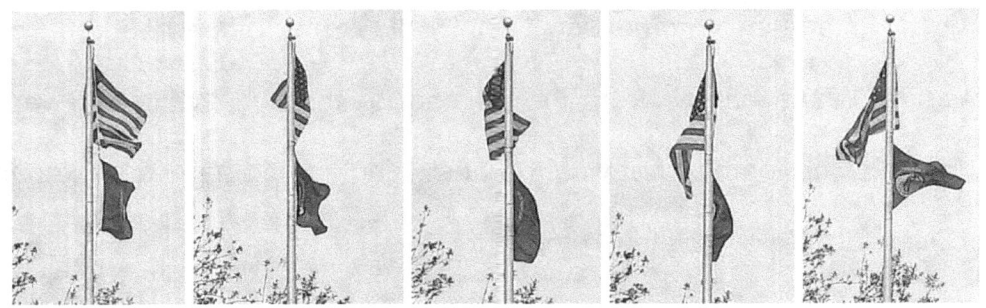

I have to walk a certain way and turn my body and my head in such a way that it doesn't impact my hair as bad. I've never seen what it looks like when I'm doing it, but co-workers have, and they're usually laughing quite noticeably about it (again, I don't get offended by any of this; I'm well aware of how silly looking it all may be, and I would undoubtedly laugh if I were watching it happen, too). Above, is an example of something that strikes a bit of---not quite terror but dread---just watching how much trees sway and how battered flags are. That tells me how windy it is outside. As of this writing, yesterday, the wind speed reached 25 MPH. I was absolutely miserable.

Co-workers at previous jobs learned very quickly my intolerance for the wind. Some would even warn me ahead-of-time that it was windy outside and to "watch out for your hair!" Again, this is actually quite comical to me, too. I often laugh along with them when this happens, but inside, I'm tormented at the thought of enduring it.

Journal Items:

12/26/2017 - wind blowing – touching my hair messing it up – very upset – don't' want to go back outside

1/19/2017 - gas station – hate how slow the pumps are – wind blowing hair – must get back in jeep

On each of the three cruises I've endured, I've had to avoid the top deck(s) because of wind. I've taken the lower, enclosed decks while friends take the top deck and meet them at the final destination. Three of us were standing just outside a deck entrance, and the wind was cutting through. One of them must have noticed the misery I was going through because he kept staring at me and motioned for us all to step indoors. I don't know what I look like when I'm experiencing the unpleasant sensation, but it probably looks like I'm being attacked by a swarm of bees.

Hypo-sensitivity

Typically, someone who is under-stimulated seeks out a thing (sometimes to excess) because he/she cannot get enough of that sensation. For me, it was the physical sensation of pressure against my hands.

Not everything touch-related was unpleasant to me. I liked the sensation of pressure. I would lie on the floor with my hand palm-side-up and deliberately place it under the rocking chair so that whenever someone was rocking in the chair, the bottom rails would roll right over my hand each time. Whomever was in it thought he/she was on a rough surface, apparently, until they would look down and notice me lying there: "get your hand out of there! You're going to hurt your hand!" I would never react or emote but would sometimes actually comply with his/her demand. When I wouldn't, the person would just get up out of the chair. That would end that.

In automobiles, I would sit in the back seat. If the window was even partially rolled-down, I would place my hand over the top edge and roll the window up---with my hand trapped---and continue cranking it up against the windowsill. Mom once pressed the UP button to roll the back window up in the car and noticed that it wasn't closing fully. She kept pressing the up button, but it wouldn't close. When she looked back, she saw my hand pinned between the window and the sill: "what are you doing!?? No wonder it wouldn't close. Get your hand out of there!" Not a word or sound from me. No reaction.

Hypo-sensitivity Versus Hyperfocus

I believe that, when I'm hyperfocused on a thing, I become numb or unaware of any physical sensation---even temperature. I've struggled with classifying this under a sensory item as opposed to a mental focus item, so it will be repeated in another chapter.

My tolerance for pain is unusual. You would think that someone as hyper-sensitive to touch as I am would have zero tolerance for pain, internal or external. This is not the case. I rarely pay attention to the fact that I'm in pain until someone mentions it or it's excruciating enough for me to actually notice. I rarely take pain medication of any kind (only once when I had an abscess tooth). I've been through a few surgeries (arterial, foot, and dental), and each time I was prescribed some kind of pain medication that I never bothered to get. I suspect that, because I'm nearly always hyperfocused on something through the day and night, I don't pay attention to the pain or the temperature---with the exception of psychosomatic pain.

Journal Item:

1/2/2017 - getting tattoo at 6 pm tonight left arm – tattoo artist asked if I needed numbing cream

Me: "no. I can tolerate pain."

Artist: "you're lucky, there."

I simply tuned-out the sensation of his needle/gun for the next hour

Many times, during winter, I've gone outside without much clothing (tank top/barefoot or shirtless) because I was focused on a specific task---so focused, in fact, that I did not pay attention to the cold. The same happens many times to me regarding the heat. I've gone into rooms and remained focused on a thing (one example would be walking into a server room and troubleshooting a performance issue and never noticing the temperature in the room having exceeded 86 degrees… which is way too hot for a server room. Someone else brought it to my attention. Only then did I realize how hot it was).

I also tend to ignore the temperature in my car and am not aware of how hot or cold it is until I have a passenger with me. It doesn't take long for him/her to roll down a window, adjust the vents, or ask for me to turn the air/heat on. In summer, I usual hear: "ooh, it's stuffy in here!" In winter, I usual hear: "doesn't your heater work?" or "it's hot as an oven in here!" Because of empathy impairment, I simply acknowledged that it was, in fact, hot, but it never occurs to me to do anything about it. It never occurs to me to see things from their perspective and to adjust the temperature accordingly---at least, not until someone tells me something, then it becomes apparent.

Journal Items:

1/3/2016 - (restaurant) friend was "chilly" at the table I chose to sit at – I wasn't feeling anything or paying attention – air not blowing on me – more focused on environment – we moved to a different table – I didn't notice the warmer temperature until he said something, and I was wearing a t-shirt the entire time – should have been cold

12/3/2016 - co-worker: "look at that. It's 83 degrees! I'm burning up!"

Me: "oh. I didn't notice… glad you said something… I usually don't pay attention."

1/12/2017 - realized I'm actually sweating and didn't notice it was hot in my office – so focused on tasks

Hyperfocus is a powerful thing. Even when I don't like being touched, if I'm hyperfocused on something, I will not notice someone touching me, much less pain or temperature. I was in the hospital, once, and the nurse was trying to take my blood while I was engaged in a conversation with 2 other people. I was so focused on what I was saying that I wasn't aware my arm was bent and stiff at a 90-degree angle---the nurse was trying to pull my arm down flat to insert the needle. My arm wouldn't budge. It wasn't until I finished what I was saying that I finally heard her saying "sir! Sir! I need to take your blood!" I apologized and lowered my arm at that point. I never felt her touch me until I broke my focus/concentration.

Another example of hyperfocus (which I detail more in another volume) happened while I was working on… something… work-related? Driving? At home? I have no idea when it happened nor HOW it happened. Couple hyperfocus with hypo-sensitivity, and you have unexplainable bruises and scratches that you don't even feel (see below photo).

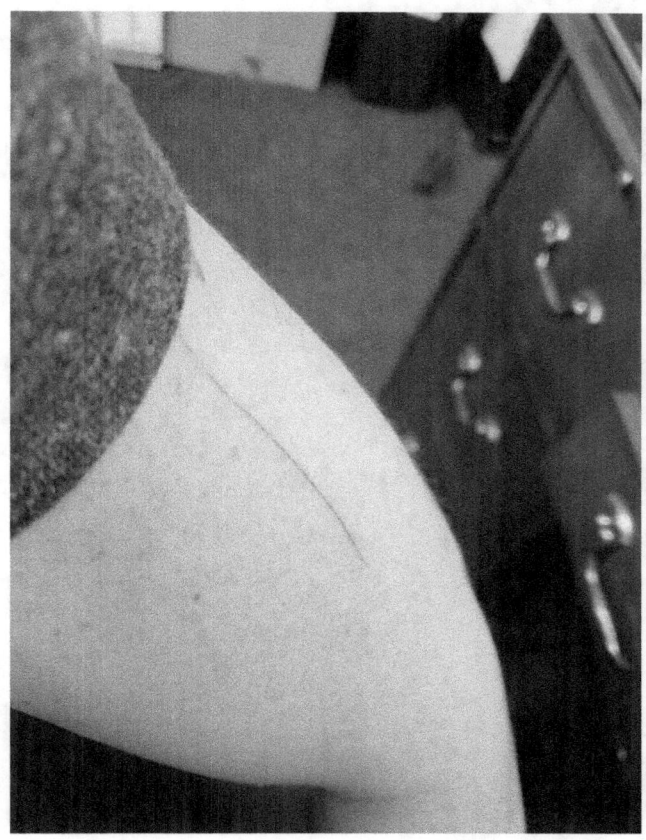

Sight

Imagine having to turn away from windows during the day or shield your eyes on a near-constant basis just to be able to function outdoors. Imagine someone shining a flashlight directly into your eyes at close range. Imagine a solar flare going-off in front of your face just because you step outside and forget to put your sunglasses on. This is what it's like for someone on The Spectrum who is hyper-sensitive to sight/bright lights. The photos, below, show what a typical day looks like to a "normal" person versus the increased intensity/hyper-sensitivity to the autistic person.

Figure 1 a normal day like this...

Figure 3 ...is more like THIS

Cameras. I used to hide my eyes or close my eyes or simply turn away if someone was taking a picture of me. Some of it was due to my poor self-image; the majority of it, however, was due to my sensitivity to the flash. Most people comment about how bright a camera flash is, but to someone on The Spectrum, a flash might as well be the sun, itself.

The picture, below left, is of me hiding behind a tiny piece of wrapping paper during Christmas at Grandma's. I was showing it off for the camera, but my eyes were closed the entire time. The funny part is this was daytime, and there was no flash on the camera. I just anticipated a flash going-off on any camera at any time. The other pictures, below, are more examples of me intentionally closing my eyes during a picture being taken or shielding my eyes from the bright outdoors or indoors (I squinted a LOT and turned my head down, looking through my eyebrows in the few photos I took).

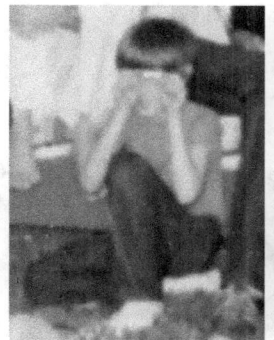 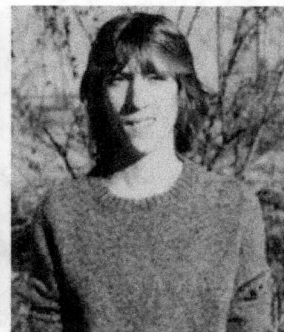 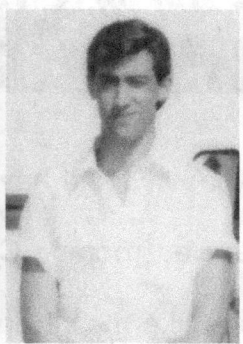 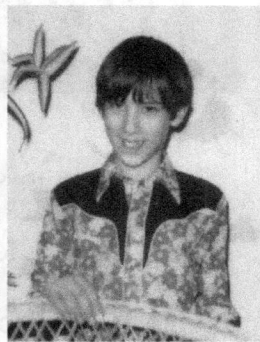

Pretty much anyone I work with or socialize with or encounter on a regular basis is used to me wearing sunglasses---even at night (if there are bright lights). Below, is a typical me photo. Once, while I was at a restaurant with two co-workers, I had a lady come up to our table, hand me a business card, and tell me she suspected I had (insert name of condition here because I cannot remember what it was called and have since lost the card) condition and suggested I contact her medical office for testing. She was convinced I had whatever it was because she had been watching me 1) never taking my sunglasses off inside the restaurant and 2) reading over the lenses (which ruled-out me using prescription sunglasses from her point-of-view, I suppose). I was quite taken-back but impressed by some stranger caring enough to extend the offer. Fortunately for that facility, I didn't waste their time on something that wasn't quite the case.

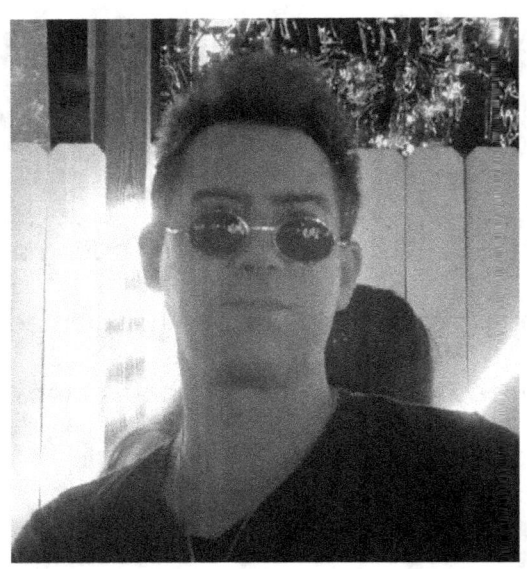

I think my life in school would have been slightly better had they allowed me to wear sunglasses in the classroom. Classrooms are extremely bright and terribly uncomfortable to someone like me. Bright offices, at least, can be controlled (usually have light dimmer switches). In one of my offices, I would not report when the bulbs would burn out so that it would remain dark enough/comfortable enough.

Journal Items:

12/26/2016 - lights too bright upstairs (at a Christmas party)

2/11/2017 - (at restaurant for lunch) sunlight... move aside (walkway) to avoid

When I was a kid, at night, street lights and head lights of any kind would drive me crazy because, every time I would blink, a stream of light would "pull" from the light source into my eyes (see the image below: picture the light 1) before blinking, 2) blinking, and 3) after blinking, and that's what it looked like); this constant sensation would stress me to the point of keeping my eyes closed most of the time while we were driving at night in the backseat of the car. Ordinarily, one might think I had some kind of eye condition or infection, but my eyes always tested 100%. I later realized that this was a normal light refraction that everyone experiences---only I was hyper-sensitive to the minute details of this occurrence and couldn't let it go for several years. Now, if I thought about it, I'd notice the effect, so I don't think about it anymore.

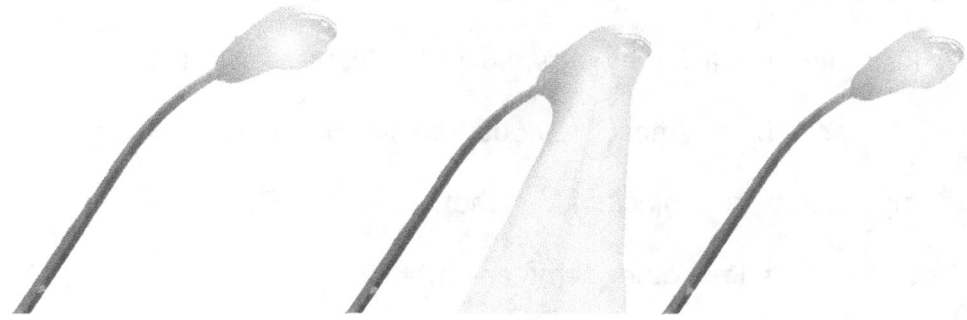

When I was little, my parents dropped me off at a friend of-the-family's house to babysit me along with her 3 other children. The son asked me to play a video game (not sure which one it was as it was not a fun game), and he noticed that I kept shielding my eyes/turning my head away from the screen every time he'd crash the space ship (very WHITE bright light would fill the screen). He started doing it on purpose to see my reaction. Little bastard.

Concerts. I both loathe and love going to concerts. See, one of my special interests is in music and vocalization. It astounds me how bands/singers can sound either just the same or completely different from their recordings, and there is no better place to test that than in a live concert. Unfortunately, there are a host of assaults on the senses for someone on The Spectrum (crowds frequently touching... interrupting intended pathways... loud, unpredictable sounds... random, pulsating, bright lights). I love looking at laser lights and spot lights when they're NOT shining directly in my eyes. Unfortunately, few concerts don't shine the lights into the audience. I've had to whip-out my sunglasses at late night concerts on more than one occasion because of it. Each time a concert ends, I tell myself that I'm never going to another concert ever again… then I end up doing it all over again.

Color. I've often told people who ask me why I "always wear black" that "color is wasted on me." It's quite true, from my perspective. I despise most colors. Black is my preferred color. My car is black (most previous vehicles were black or a grey of some kind). Most of my clothes are black. My phone, laptop, PC, notebook, briefcase, speakers, shelves, and countless other items are… black.

Why this disdain for other colors?

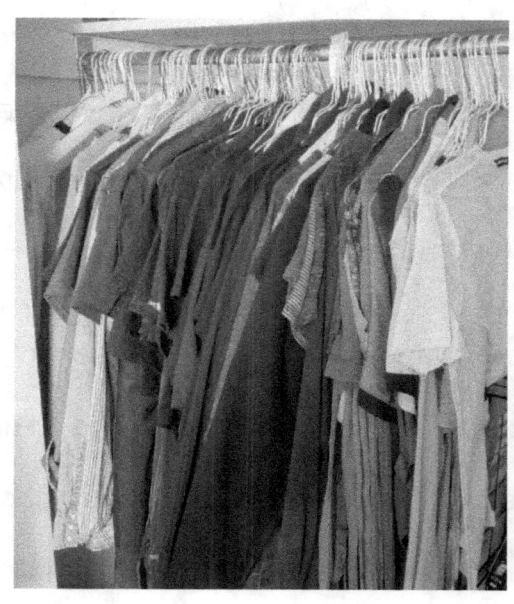

Well, I do own other colored clothes, and I force myself to wear them sometimes. As you can see from the photo above, I color coordinate my clothes in my closet. If I don't do that, I will completely overlook a shirt I would normally want to wear (my mind is looking for the specific colour as opposed to the style, so if I don't see that specific black shirt, I'll look right past it numerous times). I realize that may seem odd, but I see the color of the clothes, first, and the style, second. If I keep everything sorted by colour, then I'm fine; if I don't keep them sorted, certain clothes will be "invisible" to me. I'm not so compulsive that the sub-colors must be in a particular order (say, darkest right to lightest left), but I do keep them grouped by color. I see grey as an off-black, so grey is in my repertoire.

Someone with OCD (Obsessive-Compulsive Disorder) may freak out if the shirts are moved out of sequence or the colors mixed-up. Someone like me---who is merely compulsive---will just put the out-of-place clothing back where it "should" be without flying into a rage about it.

Once, at one of the companies I worked for, my boss played a friendly joke on me during an award nomination ceremony. He took my sunglasses and wore a black blazer with black slacks in front of all of my co-workers. Everyone immediately knew who he was impersonating. It was hilarious and is one of my fondest memories.

I've been nicknamed "the man in black" many times at work and school, and it doesn't offend me in the slightest. This is one of those preferential things I know full well draws some kind of attention (rarely negative). It could be argued by psychologists that black is an empowering color, and the reason I choose black is so that I can empower myself to go into the public. There may be a residual truth to that, but the reality is black doesn't "hurt" my eyes like orange or red or green does… and, I won't even talk about yellow or tan.

Journal Item:

2/15/2017 - bought more clothes at store – black dress pants – black pullover sweater – dark grey button-up light sweater… just cannot do colour… tried… returning tan pants – hate them

What I do find humorous is the fact I have 5 published coloring books---yet, I hate colour. Perhaps, it's my way of getting someone else to deal with coloring them in, and I don't have to.

Hypo-sensitivity

Not everything I looked at caused me displeasure. On the contrary, I sought-out certain things and was mesmerized or entranced by them, visually. My grandmother's

Christmas tree was always a highlight for me because she would dress the tree with very large glass light bulbs (multi-colored). I would lie on the couch and stare at the bulbs---the blue bulbs---study the shape and intricacy of the design... I would stare up at the ceiling and be entranced by the switching light patterns... for hours.

My parents told me that, as an infant, I would stare at the oddest things in my room. It didn't matter if it was a moving shadow or a shining reflection---I would stare at immobile objects like shoes or a bed post or the cracks in the paint on the wall or the window pane glass---I would "zoom" in on anything with a specific shape. This tendency never went away, and it's something that holds my fascination to this very day, influencing how I take photographs.

I would fixate on the key ignitions inside automobiles---especially, my aunt's because it was shaped differently compared to the others I'd seen (two tabular ends that were enormous compared to the central shaft where the keyhole was). I couldn't take my eyes off of it. I was fascinated every time I'd see someone insert the key and turn the ignition---not the act of turning on the car, but watching the key ignition twist. I would stare at odd or mundane things and would be absolutely silent (as usual).

I was always (and still am) hypnotized by waterfalls. I have no explanation for it, but as a toddler, I wandered toward a lake, saw the waterfall further ahead, and started walking toward it. I fell face-forward into the lake. My parents did not realize it happened until it was too late. Dad dove into the water and pulled me out. All I remember seeing was a bright light while looking into the water at the time. Dad said I instinctively held my breath and was "swimming like a little fish." Years later, I felt this extreme compulsion to dive off a cliff into the rapids at one of Washington D.C.'s state parks. It was the most unusual, illogical experience, but it was much like what I had experienced as a toddler. There are other examples of this, in-between the years.

Like a cat, I love looking at fast-paced, sudden visual things. I love playing against others in the swimming pool if beach balls are involved. I'll swat at anything that's in the air and anywhere near me. I love dance floors. I love watching the lights across the ceiling (or sky if it's outdoors).

Journal Item:

3/18/2017 - was sitting at a restaurant table with about 8 other guests (all acquaintances/friends) when a friend suddenly tossed a rolled-up napkin at me – caught it without looking at it or her then looked at what I caught – instantaneous reaction – like a cat.

Sound

Sound is another big one for me as I'm hyper-sensitive to certain sounds and pitches. Some, I can ignore; others, I cannot and will avoid at all costs. I will say that my ability to tune-out unpleasant sounds has improved, considerably, over the years. My hearing is particularly tuned to high pitched sounds.

Journal Item:

9/14/2015 - work – buzzing sound – co-workers couldn't hear it but I could – asked if our facilities tech could help find/fix it – thought it was in the air vent – ended up coming from the back of an old monitor while it was plugged in

Loud voices and loud vehicles, primarily, would send me into a locked-up state, as a kid.

I was rarely happy to see my other relatives come over to visit during holidays because they were very LOUD---abrasive, intrusive voices and personalities. They knew I was "shy" and didn't want to interact, so they would single me out because of it. They were not abusive, by any means, but they could certainly sense I was not like the rest of them. I would try to hide and remain reclusive, but there were few places to hide in Grandma's small house.

As a kid, I refused to play with any toy that made clicking sounds. These were usually battery-operated or had some kind of action lever that needed to be pushed to move an arm or leg or head. I hated this. I liked all parts to be free moving so that I had full control over them, so I would usually wear the clicking mechanism down to make it stop.

Journal Item:

1/19/2017 - sound of my clanging necklace aggravating me (metal clanging against metal) – must fix it – remove extra piece from necklace – make sound stop

Loud motorcycles seemed to be more common back then when I was a kid, so I had to endure that noise. I actually liked motorcycles and, surprisingly, I enjoyed riding on ours with my parents. I hated the helmet more than you can imagine (ref. touch), but I equally hated the breeze while riding, too. I would stand far away from dirt bikes because they were the loudest. I actually owned two motorcycles over the years and have forced myself to endure the blowing sensation out of sheer will until I simply could no longer bare it. My riding trips were not really pleasant and quite brief. I did enjoy riding a motorcycle in the desert in Phoenix, Arizona because I could, at least, ride it slow and control the sensation.

Hot air balloons terrified me for three reasons: 1) they were huge, 2) the sight of the burner, and 3) the sound of the burner. Growing up in Albuquerque (hosts the largest hot air balloon fiesta in The United States), every October hot air balloons were all over the place: on the ground, pulled behind vehicles on trailers, and in the sky. I loved looking at them in the sky and found it difficult to NOT look at them seemingly suspended up there like pins in cushions---or, more relatedly---like bigger versions of Grand Ma's Christmas Tree bulbs that I was so entranced with at the time. My parents made the mistake of taking me to the actual fiesta grounds when I was about 5 or 7 years-old. They carried me up to a balloon that was filling-up, and I zeroed-in on the flame, but it was the sound of the burner that caused me to lose it. I broke out in a screeching wail, and Mom had to take me back up the grassy hill. I watched Dad continue walking toward it and started screaming for him to stop (I thought the balloon was going to hurt him). I've never been close to a balloon since. You see, dogs and cats go through the same freak-out. Their senses are tuned-in much like an autistic's is. The result is the same: panic.

Thunder. I actually love the sound of thunder, but the first time I hear it, I stiffen-up briefly. It's easier to deal with natural sounds since there is little that can be done to avoid them. The sound of firecrackers is far worse, and I fully understand why cats and dogs scramble under tables and hide in closets because of them.

To me, though, the sound of shrilling alarms and sirens are the absolute worst sound of them all. I'll never understand why people will stop what they're doing to LOOK up at an ambulance or firetruck passing by once they hear the siren---what's the point? I never do. I recognize the sound, and I know they're heading somewhere.

One of the most notable meltdowns I experienced was at an indoor movie theater. I was about 8 years-old. I lasted into the first 15 minutes of the movie (King Kong) before I absolutely lost it. I was screaming and covering my ears and crying. My parents had to carry me out of the theater and take me home. I kept saying that it was "too loud! Too loud!" No one else was complaining, though. I remember glancing up at the crowded theater, and most of the people seated around us were staring at me---straight-faced. Why weren't THEIR ears hurting? Why weren't THEY crying and leaving? Why was it only ME?

The furnace. Grandma had an old gas furnace that was in the adjoining front room behind a very large, wooden door. I could hear it kick-on, and that was alerting enough as it was, but when someone would open the door, I would absolutely freak OUT. I would lose it. Part of it was visual in seeing this erupting blue flame coming out of dark twisted metal; most of it, though, was hearing the thunderous sound of the flame. Combine the two, and you had a kid with furnace-phobia (yes, I just made that word up). My parents and Grandma tried to get me to get over my fear of that furnace, but it never worked. I simply envisioned a monster in there---not unlike a dragon or demon. I gave it a name: "Dolf-a-On." I have no idea where that name came from, but it stuck for years.

Speaking of reciprocation, another thing I do is rarely-if-ever turn and look in the direction of any sudden noise (like most people tend to do). I've been in restaurants and other establishments where a dish falls and breaks or someone falls from a stool or trips or someone spills something on the floor---I almost never bother to look in that direction because… why? Why do that when it was obvious from hearing the recognizable sound. If a person has never heard that sound before (e.g. an infant or young toddler), then I can understand why he/she would look to see what the source of the sound might be for future reference. I don't bother reacting in that manner, and I'll be one of the very few people in a public place that continues what he was already doing before the sudden noise was created.

Journal Items:

1991 - Phoenix, AZ - encountered numerous Black Widow spiders – they lived in the tool shed next to the house – I could HEAR them climbing on their webs – put my hand through their webs by accident several times – petrified to go near that shed or under cars.... they seemed to be everywhere - began studying everything about them as a result

1/3/2016 - (restaurant) heard high pitched crash/metal bang way in the back... did not react... paying more attention to how I zone-in on sounds... realized I cock my head or turn head funny when focused on listening... probably looks strange

Power tools. It's astounding to me how difficult it is to escape power tools through one's life. The first time I heard Grand Pa's drills or saws, I lost it. I could NOT handle that sound. They were loud, shrilling, and invasive. Hearing them is like feeling daggers pierce the skin---I can't describe it any better than that. I was forced to take a shop class in Middle School---once---and I never touched any of the power tools. We had to switch me out of that class because I was definitely going to fail it, and I refused to get near the workbenches. The free tools (hammers, hand saws, etc.) were perfectly fine, and I still use them to this day. The teacher---like most back then---was unsympathetic and thought I was being a sissy about it. If I could have switched places with him just for 5 minutes so that he could have experienced the torture, he would have been a much more understanding person as a result.

Up until 2015, I had never ventured out of this country. I did a bit of traveling with some folks over the years (rarely by my own choice; I would usually just follow along because it seemed like an interesting thing to experience). On my second cruise (ship), we left port during a storm, so the ship was rocking heavily. I don't get sea sick, so the motion didn't bother me whatsoever (perhaps, it's my hypofocus being a strength, in this case). What did bother me, however, was the continuous clinking and clanking of the metal objects in the cabin. I had little-to-no sleep that first night because of it, and I was useless the next day, as a result. That was a miserable experience. I primarily use a fan at night for "white noise" to drown-out all other sounds, and that was a luxury I didn't have on this particular cruise.

Journal Items:

1/12/2017 - woke up – fixated on sound of pillow against left ear – feathers inside – deafening – move on to back – fine after changing positions – can't hear feathers inside now

1/12/2017 - sound of chair in office at work – squeaks every time I take a breath – had to swap out with quiet chair - better

1/23/2017 - could not sleep - clang ng of coat hangers – light bulb loose in fixture in bathroom keeps rolling back-and-forth – closet door keeps clinking – creaking of cabin walls (while on a cruise during a storm at sea)

1/24/2017 - no white noise (fan) – listened counted every sound – counted number of occurrences and in-between each occurrence – realized I have headphones in bag – after putting them on was able to sleep just fine rest of night (2nd day on cruise during storm at sea)

Crying babies. Most people don't like the sound of screaming babies unless it's their own. Airplanes and restaurants and theaters are the worse-case environments for babies to start screaming. I bring headphones and will put them on as quickly as possible to avoid the unpleasant sound. When I don't have that coping mechanism available, it becomes torturous.

Journal Item:

2/11/2017 - (at restaurant for lunch) screaming baby… agitating… walking much quicker down aisle to get as far away as possible

Hypo-sensitivity

I loved loud music (and still do). In the interest of keeping my hearing excellent, I only do it in spurts and only with specific songs, but I did/do seek out loud music. In fact, that is the only thing, sound-wise, that I seek out. I was never one of those kids who kept playing with an object just to hear the sound it made, over-and-over (there are some who do).

Another thing I love to do is listen-in on other conversations at nearby tables when I'm in a restaurant or coffee shop or other public places. Why? I do not know. Perhaps, I'm simply eavesdropping. Perhaps, in my mind, because everyone is in a public place, we're all part of the same interactive experience, and their conversations are my conversations. I may never know why I do this.

Sound

Since childhood and through my teen years, my sense of smell was quite acute, but I never really paid much attention to it. I wouldn't get overloaded from smell, thankfully, as I had enough to contend with. To this day, I will detect a smell, cock my head (like a dog), analyze it, but continue with my task, undisturbed. Essentially, my sense of smell is quite attuned, but I try to purposely ignore it whenever possible.

Oddly enough, I lost my sense of smell between 1990 and 2008.

I say I lost my sense of smell, but it was exceedingly dulled-down. I came down with Valley Fever (a unique fungal infection in the lungs that caused a strain of pneumonia) in Phoenix, AZ. It took me a month and-a-half to recover from it, but after it was gone, I had minor scar tissue on my lung, and my sense of smell had all but gone away. As unusual an occurrence that was, I actually didn't miss smelling things.

In 2008, my sense of smell came back. I have no idea why or how. I don't know how much of it was mental versus physical, much less any possible action that may have triggered it. One day, I started smelling everything near me as if it was all brand new. It was a surprisingly pleasant experience, and I now don't take it for granted as much as I used to.

Hypo-sensitivity

Although, I never sought out specific smells, I did use smell as a memory time capsule of sorts. The moment I would smell something---if I'd smelled it before---it would trigger an instant memory and emotion from that moment. Having researched memory, I learned that smell can trigger memory faster than any other sense. I suppose I used it in a slightly different manner than most folks. I would smell a leather jacket so that I could recall specific memories (my teens) of when I wore a leather jacket, years prior.

I did enjoy the smell of playdough and glue.

As a kid, I sought-out the smell of motorcycle display rooms (I mentioned owning two of them, earlier). I don't know if it was the smell of the oil or the exposed engines or the new machines, but I do remember looking forward to going to motorcycle dealerships just to experience that smell.

When I moved to Louisville in 2000, I immediately picked-up a strong scent that I never smelled in any other city. Apparently, it was the smell of the distilleries in the region (since Louisville, KY is known for its bourbon), and I loved going outside, especially in mornings when the air was still free from typical city smells, just to pick-up on the "Louisville scent." Sadly, the smell is all but gone since many distilleries have closed up, relocated out-of-town, or modified their environments so that not as much escapes the facilities----quite frankly, I do not know why the smell is essentially gone, now.

Apart from that, my notes on smell are minimal.

Taste

As little impact smell has on me, taste has even less impact. I suppose I do find specific things may taste good or bad---like anyone else---but, I don't really pay much attention to that fact. If I'm eating something, it's in my preference list for a reason which is usually because the texture is fine, it looks fine, and it fits with my routine (specific eating establishments I go to on a scheduled basis – see my other chapter on restrictive routine/sameness).

I did enjoy eating rose pedals and glue, for some reason. I guess I enjoyed the taste.

Apart from that, I have little to add here.

Chapter Conclusion

Ordinarily, someone on The Spectrum may or may not be able to develop the self, depending on how severe/what degree it is for him/her. I was fortunate to have a drive to overcome obstacles---not be victimized by them. I attained an Associate's Degree in Criminal Justice after 4 years; I attained a Bachelor's Degree in Information Technology after 1.5 years; I attained a Master's Degree in Managing Information Technology after 1.5 years; I'm (as of this writing) pursuing a PhD in Information Technology. The point to my sharing all of this is that anything can be overcome---albeit, with significant effort.

It's overwhelming as a child. It's depressing as a teen. It's agitating as an adult. It CAN be WORKED with.

All of these years, all of these struggles, all of these accomplishments, all of these strengths had led me to the source of it all. I am different. I know why, now. I was singled-out and ostracized because of that difference. I was accepted and supported because of that difference. I am unique. I am the same. I am a person… just like you.

ROUTINES, COMPULSIVENESS, AND RESTRICTED SPECIAL INTERESTS

Having a routine is having a sense of sameness. Having a routine creates a sense of that which has already been discovered, is already known, and poses no risks of failure, embarrassment, or any other awkward association. It's for this very reason autistic persons stick to routines---and are quite adamant about not altering them very much else a meltdown of some kind may occur.

The DSM-V defines it as restricted, repetitive patterns of behaviour, interests, or activities, as manifested by at least two of the following, currently or by history [1]:

- Stereotyped or repetitive motor movements, use of objects, or speech

- Insistence on sameness, inflexible adherence to routines, or ritualized patterns of verbal or nonverbal behaviour

- Highly restricted, fixated interests that are abnormal in intensity or focus

- Hyper- or hypo-reactivity to sensory input or unusual interest in sensory aspects of the environment

In this chapter, I'm focusing on the first two items.

Routines are static, non-changing patterns of behaviour. The best way to understand the concept of routines in the autistic mind is to think of routes. People like me prefer very specific, consistent routes in everything we do and everywhere we go. Something that is introduced that breaks the routine can completely throw us off-balance (mentally and even physically in regards to clumsiness). I've had some days where my routine was interrupted, and I couldn't reset myself for several hours afterwards. It's that important to us. The outsider may witness this ritualistic behaviour we exhibit and simply think we're "creatures of habit" or just like things "being consistent." Those are not untrue statements, but they are terrifically under-stated in terms of importance to us.

Again, having preferences is nothing unusual for a "normal" person or someone on The Spectrum. What is different is how consistent we are about maintaining the routine and what happens when we don't. Being territorial, also, is a common trait for those on The Spectrum. Some will go into a mild-to-severe meltdown if routines are broken. Fortunately, I'm not that bad about it, but it does affect me in other ways.

Unfortunately (or, thankfully?), self-medicating becomes a routine. Because sleep is often a victim of a mind that does not turn off, naturally, I have to resort to a specific brand of cold/flu medicine. I take it each-and-every single night 20 minutes before I anticipate going to sleep. I take it, take whatever medication I need to for the night, head upstairs and lie down in bed and watch TV. This is my nightly ritual. Once the cold/flu medicine kicks-in, I go unconscious and rarely dream (well, recall dreaming, that is). If I do not stick to this routine, I will wake up around 4:00 A.M. (within that hour) with my mind replaying every social event I may have engaged in, earlier that day, or problem-solving something I've been troubleshooting, or rehearsing conversations I may or may not have later that day.

Breaking a routine can have certain consequences, so adhering to the routine--- no matter what---creates the appearance of being aloof:

Journal Item:

3/27/2017 - female at the gas pump parallel to mine forgot to put her pump handle/hose away/take out of her vehicle – she drove away and snapped the hose off – then slammed brakes... I did not stay – I had to get to the gym/lunch – this was not part of the plan – I did not react/emote – I continued filling my tank and left

My sleep schedule is very strict---even on trips: I must have exactly 7 hours of sleep – not 8 – not 6, otherwise my next day will be miserable (low energy/ "off" timing/ lack of focus)

My getting ready routine would be consistent for years at-a-time, depending on the variables and environment. Here is a sample routine in the 90's:

- go to sink - turn on hot water - get towel/fold onto sink ledge - lean on towel with both hands under the hot water - stand there for 10 to 15 minutes - stick head under faucet - wash hair with specific brand shampoo/conditioner (conditioner has to be applied after at least 5 min. and soak for 5 min.) - entire duration can last 20 to 30 minutes JUST to wash hair

- soak hair in towel for 10 to 15 min. - towel dry hair

- wait 5 min. - hair dryer + specific brand hairspray

- apply specific brand coconut butter face cream

- check - double-check mirrors for imperfections

- yell back at whomever is yelling at me to "hurry up!!!"

- entire duration: 2hrs

Anyone wanting me to go somewhere with him/her HAD to give me a 2 hour warning ahead-of-time with not much variation in this routine through the 2000s. I had to alter some things due to work start times and residence environment + roommates and cutting my hair short.

I order the same things and do not deviate for very long periods of time. If I do deviate, I remain screwed-up with my routine out-of-sync, an instant dislike for the new thing I've just tried, and an instant desire to return to the previous item I was ordering. There are some things I simply never deviate from.

Some retail establishments absolutely love someone like me because I'm highly predictable. I'm the perfect data mining subject (for online purchases) because I buy things in groupings or modes---which create easily forecastable patterns. It's very easy to gather and interpret statistics from someone as compulsive as me.

My threshold (level of tolerance) is quite high, regarding my eating habits. When I was younger, my parents or grandma would dictate what I had for dinner; school would dictate what I had for lunch. When I became more independent, my ordering habits slipped back into a compulsive state that had always been there, and I remain "stuck" in an ordering routine that doesn't change for months at-a-time. I have examples in the later eating and ordering chapter.

I have a specific locker at my gym that I use (2nd from left, bottom row, near mirror). The gym doesn't allow assigned lockers, unfortunately, and I won't use any random available locker near it---I do have a secondary locker on the other side of the room that I will use if I have to. It aggravates me when someone is already using it before I get there. I push the bench out of the way so that no one else will be tempted to sit near my locker while I'm getting dressed.

Here is another example of sameness. I will wear the same clothes, boots, use the same things until they are no longer usable. In this example, I go through boots rather quickly (a pair-per-year) because of the way I walk in them---that stiff, robot-like, hard walk where I don't redistribute my weight very well and apply far too much pressure while walking. As a result, my boots wear down rather quickly.

Even if there are holes in the soles and water seeps in when it's raining, I still wear them. This particular pair (shown on the left) wasn't thrown away until the heel completely came off of the left boot.

I rarely care how they look. It's the fact that they are "just right."

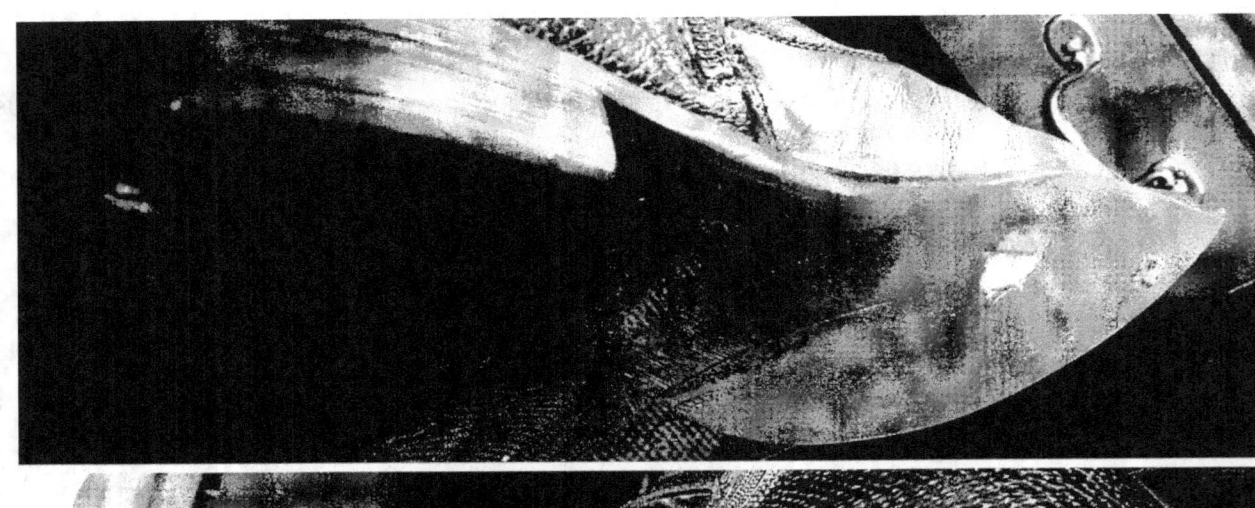

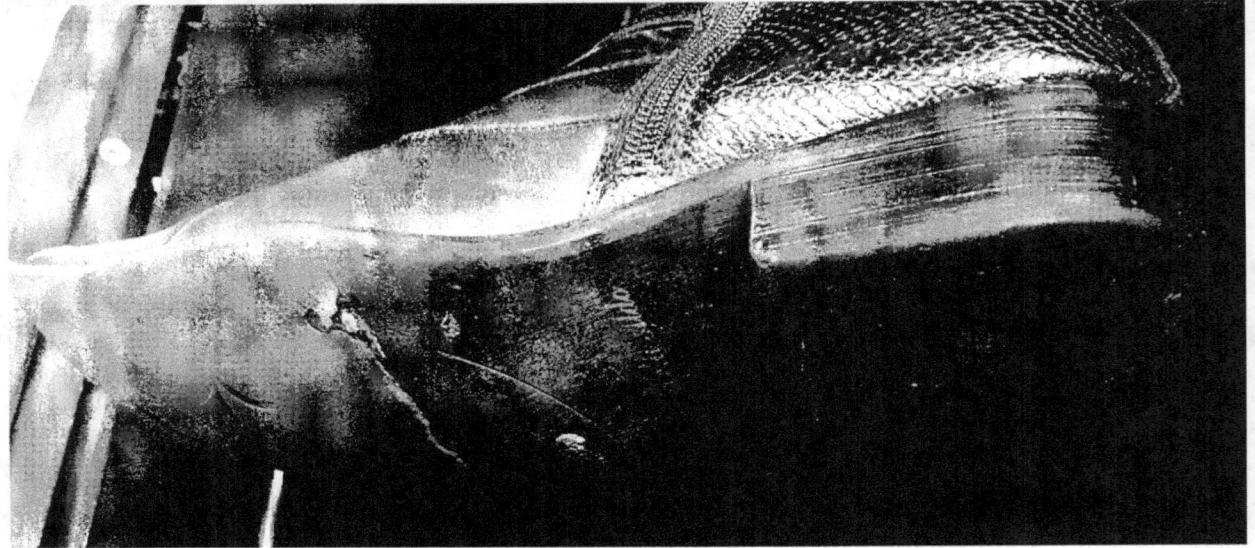

My disdain for certain colors in clothing, cars, laptops, PCs, and any other material object was mentioned in an earlier chapter, but the necessity for sameness in color preference falls-in, here, too. I compulsively wear black and grey colors and only force myself to wear blue or pink when necessary.

Having rehearsed, preemptive responses helps folks like me avoid saying something awkward or experience that awkward pause. Here is my list of rehearsed responses:

Cool	That kicks ass
Will do	I love it
Can do	Just fine. How are you?
OK	Doing well. How are you?
YES/NO	Thank you.
Hey, how are you doing?	Interesting.
Good (morning, afternoon)	

Journal Items:

3/27/2017 - coffee shop – I messed up greetings with new barista... she said "hey there." Me: "just fi---how are you?" I caught myself before saying "just fine. How are you?"

3/27/2017 - restaurant - I Don't feel nervous or anxious.... took a while to pick out a table.... back not to door.... back not to crowd.... can see TVs on wall.... but feeling muscle ache suddenly in lower back 5 min. later

4/5/2017 - coffee shop - I came up to 2nd register/barista – he already had my order keyed-in. The customer next to me at 1st register/barista said: "wow, you didn't even have to open your mouth."

I caught myself standing in the same spot inside the same coffee shop I frequent every morning of every weekday, one day. I began to notice I do this everywhere I go--- same side, same chair, same corner, same bench, same pathway, same.... This is the very essence of restricted routine and compulsiveness. In the case of the photo, below, I took of myself in 2016, I stand in the EXACT spot. I didn't believe I was really THAT compulsive until I took photos of where I stood for several days at-a-time. As always, I require visual and empirical proof of a thing and not just casual observation.

Why stand in the same spot each morning? It's the same answer for why I walk the same path in the same store each morning: it's a known variable to me; it's safe; I have little likelihood of tripping over something unforeseen or interrupting my efficiency in getting out of the building as quickly as possible.

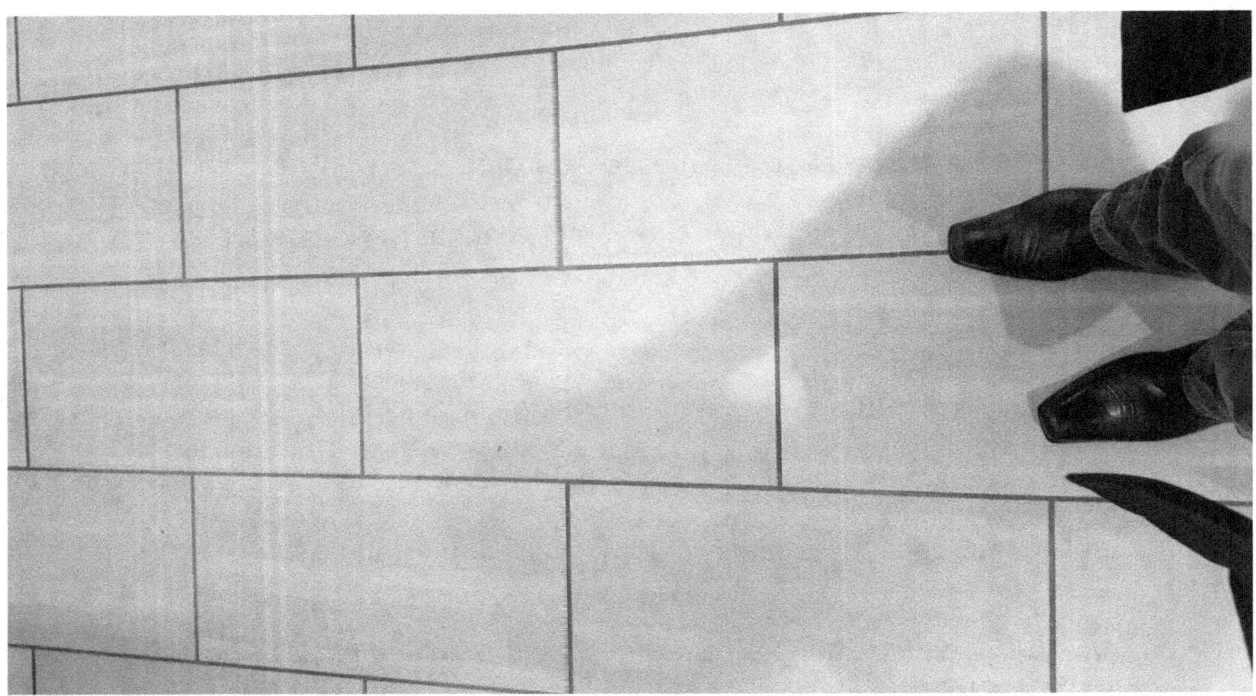

The below example is a data capture I did involving my strict listening habits. I knew my entire life that I would only listen to a specific genre at-a-time and would rarely mix genres. I didn't know how long that routine would last, duration-wise. I pulled the data from my online streaming service (purchase history) and was able to group everything according to average, total, and instances, capturing my threshold.

Music Listening History		
Duration (yrs.)	4.9	6/2012 to 7/2017
AVG Days Per-Genre (Threshold)	**30**	Conclusion: *on average*, I remain "locked" into one music genre for 30 days before switching to a different music genre. It takes me an *average* of 2 days to switch between "locked" genres. This means I do not typically deviate while I'm "locked" into a music genre..... until it's time to switch.
AVG Gap Between Genres (days)	2	
Genres (general)	14	
Genres (distinct)	24	

Average Duration (days) per-Genre		Total Duration (days) per-Genre		Instances per-Genre	
synth	53	rock	632	rock	22
new wave	42	club	243	club	10
Christmas	36	Christmas	179	unknown	7
oldies	33	new wave	127	CCM	6
rock	29	CCM	109	Christmas	5
soundtracks	26	country	70	new wave	3
club	24	unknown	69	country	3
country	23	oldies	65	indie	3
new age	22	indie	56	oldies	2
big band	21	synth	53	soundtracks	2
indie	19	soundtracks	52	classical	2
CCM	18	classical	35	synth	1
classical	18	new age	22	new age	1
unknown	10	big band	21	big band	1

I don't just listen to the music. I'm very much hooked on vocals. I listen-in on vocal pitch, timbre, projection, range, and study other aspects of vocalization such as key and octave. I have no interest in being a singer, personally, but it is a special interest which means I must study everything about it. I've purchased singing courses and an electric piano---just so I can better associate vocals to the keys of a piano. There are specific singers (male and female) who I instantly gravitate toward and collect any recorded or live productions they may have available. I'm fixated by tenor, baritone, soprano, alto, etc. and love holding my vocal frequency app up to various singers to watch how their pitch registers.

Below, is a photo of the electric piano I purchased:

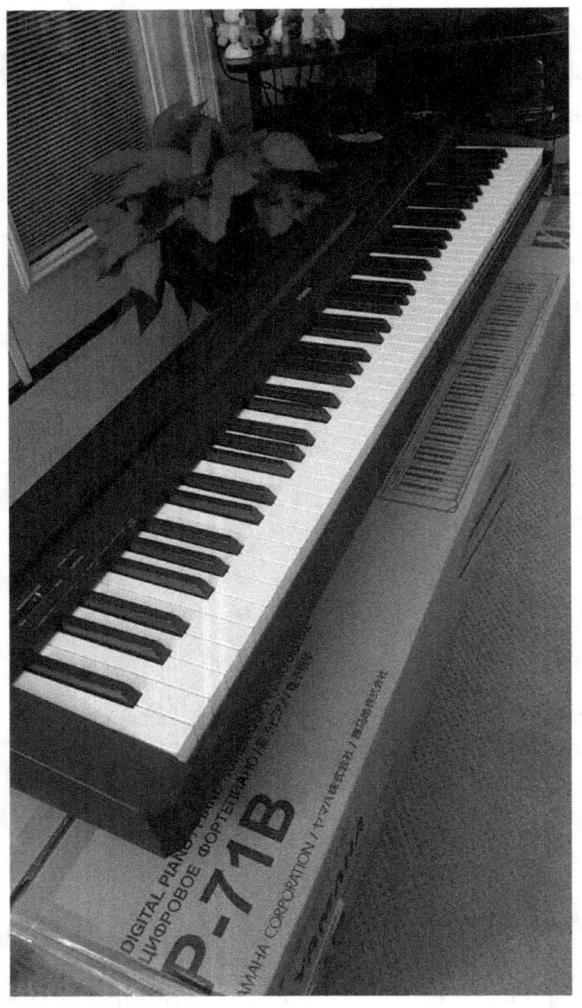

That being said, I'm also very attuned to the actual music, itself, and find myself entranced by 80's electronica music (no vocals), in particular, and have vast collections of it from various artists.

I memorize the track order of albums (depending on how they are arranged or sorted). Especially before digital music, if a song scratched/skipped, it would completely lock me up (again, it's a routine/order thing), and I would memorize the exact spot it would skip (or break or cut-out); to this day, even though I listen exclusively to digital music, I still remember and anticipate the spot on certain songs that used to skip/break.

At work and any place I frequent, I have my primary and secondary parking spots. This isn't always an easy thing to maintain as random people have no clue the spot they're parking in is actually mine. Do I get upset if someone parks in my spot? YEP. Do I become rude and confrontational about it? NOPE. I will be annoyed, but I will park in a different, secondary spot. The moment mine becomes available, however, I claim it.

The two photos, below, were taken exactly one year apart from each other. I traded my jeep in for a small sports car. That's all that changed. I still park in the same spot, no matter how empty the lot may be. When I took the latest pic (bottom left), there were no cars in the lot. Even though I could have parked closer to the door, I didn't.

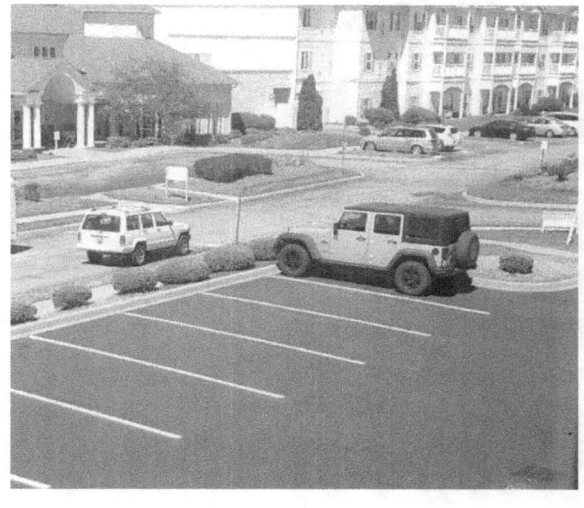 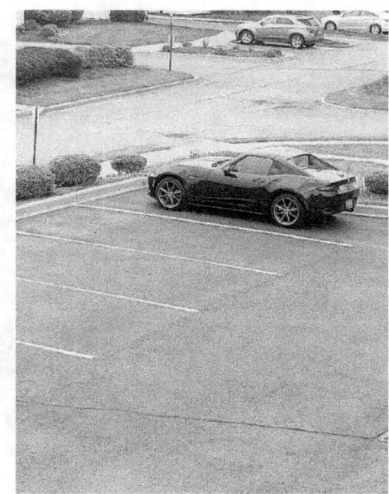

My tendency to do the same thing (repetition) and stick with it (sameness) doesn't take much planning or preparation. In fact, one might say it's instinctual since it's a tendency I was born with. My tendency is to seek out corners---like I used to do in school with the desks I would choose to sit in.

It's near-impossible to not encounter a new, unpredictable situation or environment. What is possible is quickly adopting a new routine by adapting to a new place to stand or walk through/to or a new food item to order off a new menu. Once something works--- that's it---there is no deviating from that point-forward.

Routines are especially evident while driving. I have very specific routes I take and have secondary (fallback) routes ready in case an accident or other exigent circumstance interferes with the primary route. Below, is a snapshot of the primary and START OF DAY and END OF DAY routes I took for nearly 6 years:

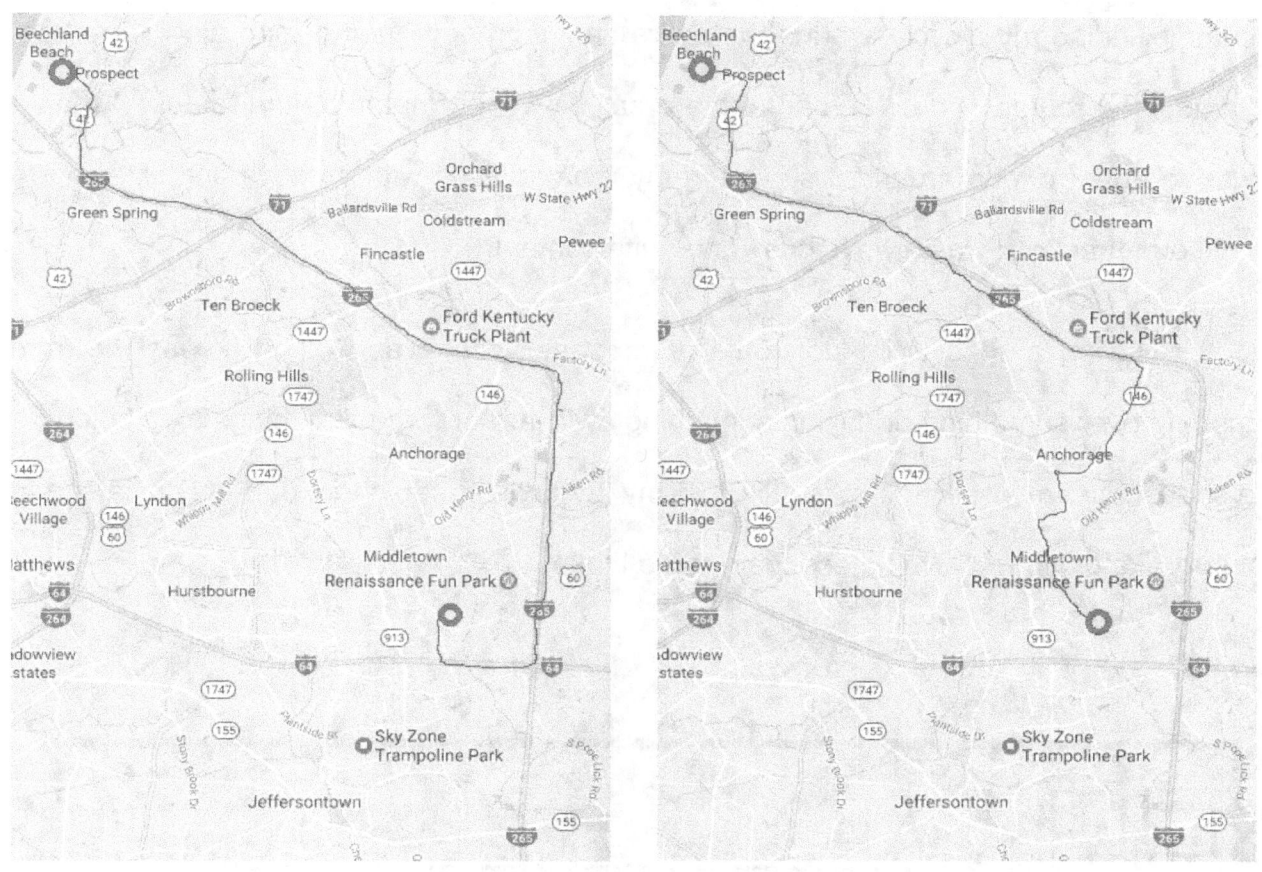

Below, is a snapshot of my LUNCH route for nearly 6 years:

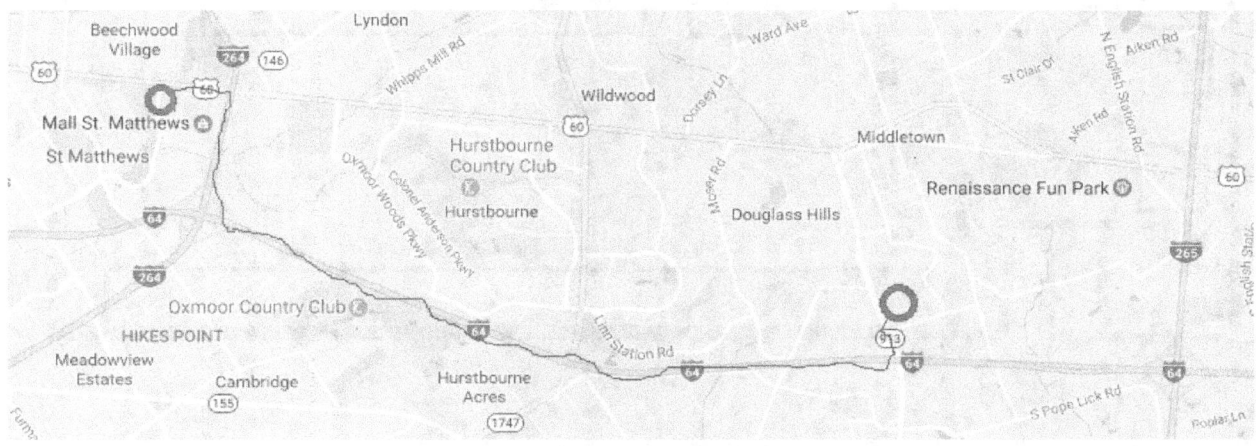

During my 6th Grade year, I had no friends (typical), and I would spend the entire summer riding my bicycle around the entire neighborhood, memorizing all of the street names and routes. I drew a map of the area. I was fascinated by the routes. When it was too dark to ride around, I stayed in my room playing with my toys and listening to my soundtracks. I was always busy and quite content.

Having a specific interior route is important to me, as well. It keeps me from tripping over something or saying something awkward or forgetting things or… below, is a snapshot of my walking routine INSIDE my favourite coffee shop. I rarely deviate, and if I do, like driving, I have a secondary route I take.

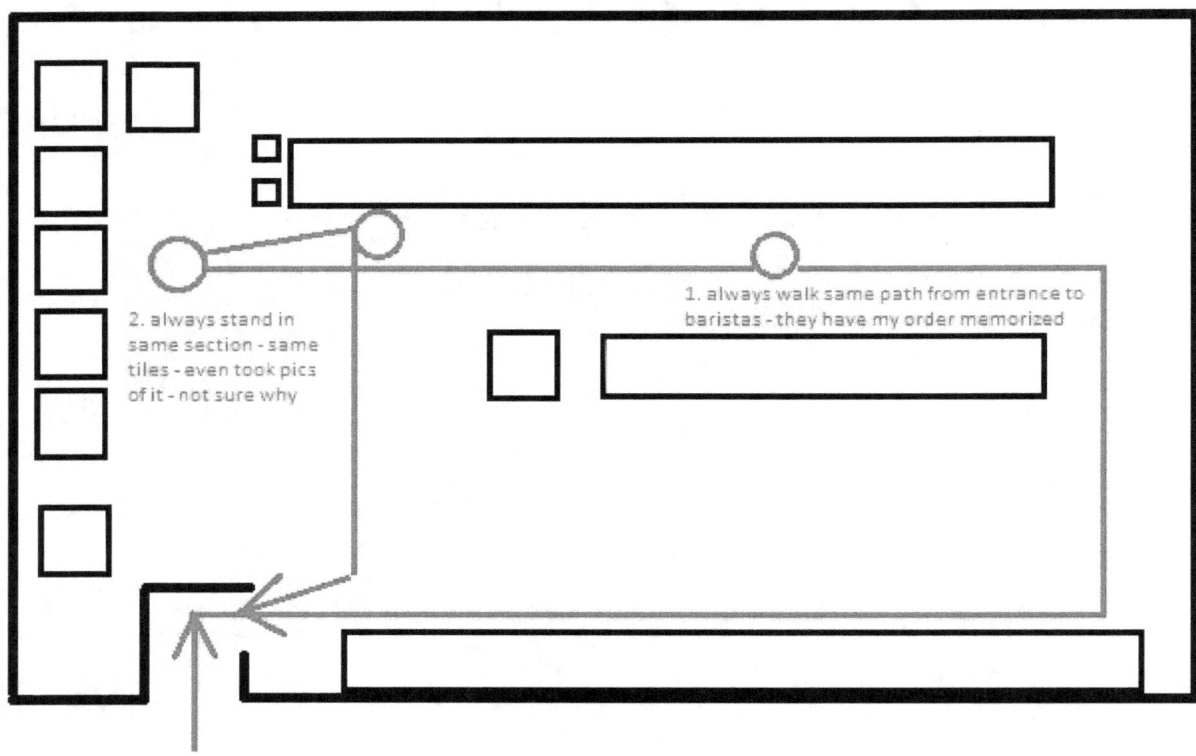

Regarding the same coffee shop, I do have a secondary one I go to at another part of the city. Below, is a graph of a study I conducted on myself (using my credit card previous purchase history) that shows how often I frequent the same store and on which days of the week.

It shows a fairly consistent routine in the 80 to 90 day period per each weekday.

Weekends are much lower in frequency because my routine changes on weekends (typically stay home in the mornings, but there are specific things I eat/drink, routinely, there).

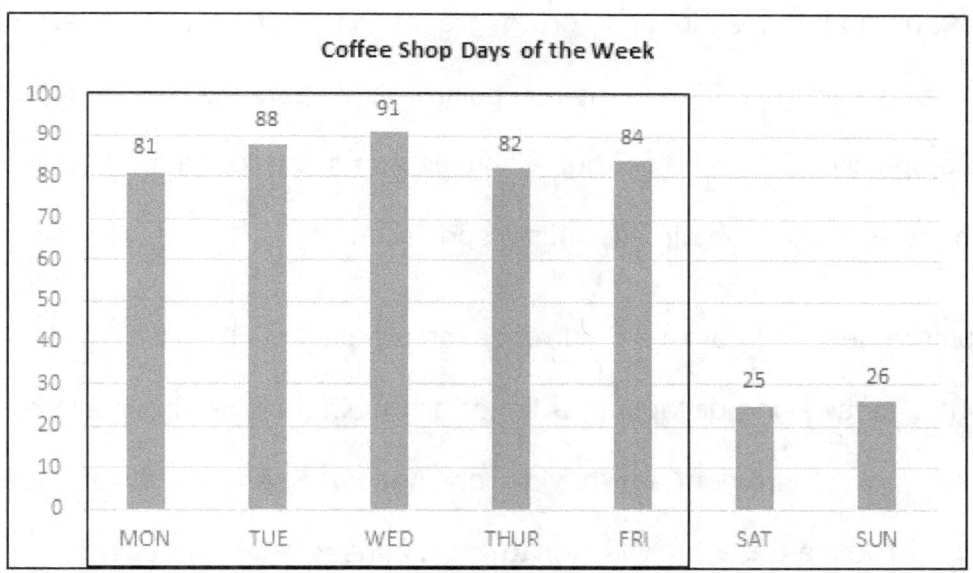

Regarding the same coffee shop, I do have a secondary one I go to at another part of the city. Below, is a graph of a study I conducted on myself (using my credit card previous purchase history) that shows how often I frequent the same store and on which days of the week.

It shows a fairly consistent routine in the 80-to-90-day period per each weekday.

Weekends are much lower in frequency because my routine changes on weekends (typically stay home in the mornings, but there are specific things I eat/drink, routinely, there).

Repetition

Repetition is a key component to the autistic brain. In some ways, it's the brain getting "stuck" into a cyclical pattern that does not end until it's time to end. In other ways, it's a manifestation of something so enjoyable/method of relief that it's difficult to stop doing the act.

There are many descriptions for the repetitious act (aka "perseveration" or "compulsiveness"). I prefer the term, compulsiveness, personally. It is part of the Obsessive-Compulsive Disorder title, but it isn't just restricted to that particular disorder. Compulsiveness also exists within the autism spectrum.

Compulsiveness is state of recurrence or repetition. It can involve repetitive motor motions (like swaying or tapping a finger or rubbing a face) or repetitive choices and practices. A requirement for having an Autism Spectrum Disorder is being compulsive and routine-based. It is not to be confused with Obsessive-Compulsive Disorder as that is its own, distinct diagnosis. Many people, I find, misuse the term, "OCD," and are describing a compulsive act versus an obsessive-compulsive one. Having an obsession is having something undesirable (such as a fear of germs or being dirty) that may lead into a compulsive behaviour to avoid that obsession. Compulsive behaviour---in the autistic mind---is typically a very pleasant, safe, desirable state of being. Another way of understanding the concept of being compulsive is using the word, sameness, which I'm quite fond of. "Addiction" is also a similar word to describe compulsion. As with "OCD", I tend to misuse the word "habit" at times. A habit is something that can be interrupted. A compulsion, on the other hand, cannot be interrupted without some sort of consequence (even a minor one). I tend to combine routine with compulsiveness because they are linked.

I order the SAME coffee drink and have been doing so since 2006 when I discovered I could substitute dairy for soy. My order: "I'll have a grande peppermint white mocha with soy and no whip." Because of my sameness, the coffee shop employees already know to ring my order up before I have to open my mouth. Sometimes, I may even add a chocolate chip cookie, but it isn't often.

My current lunch order consists of 2 Extra Crispy Chicken Breasts + bottled water. I've been on this routine since May 2017 with very little deviation or alteration. As with routines, I always have a backup/Go To selection, but this is where I will be at for several more months, possibly.

Below, is a capture of my previous eating routine and its duration:

1988	ramen noodles + uncle ben's boiling bag rice	Lunch
1989	ramen noodles + uncle ben's boiling bag rice	lunch
1990	ramen noodles + uncle ben's boiling bag rice	lunch
1990	rarely if ever ate lunch - would wait until dinner	lunch
2000	rarely if ever ate lunch - would wait until dinner	lunch
2000	Pizza (cheese + pepperoni) + med coke	lunch
2001	Pizza (cheese + pepperoni) + med coke	lunch
2003	Pizza (cheese + pepperoni) + med coke	lunch
2004	various (due to co-worker lunches)	lunch
2005	various (due to co-worker lunches)	lunch
2006	various (due to co-worker lunches)	lunch
2007	various (due to co-worker lunches)	lunch
2007	Fast food (crispy chicken sandwich + potato cake + med coke)	lunch
	Fast food (chicken sandwich + sm fries + sm coke)	
	Fast food (spicy chicken sandwich + med coke)	
2008	Fast food (buffalo chicken strips + med coke)	lunch
	Fast food (chicken sandwich + sm fries + sm coke)	
	Fast food (spicy chicken sandwich + med coke)	
2009	Fast food (12in or 6in spicy Italian + bbq chips or pnt btr cookie + sm coke)	lunch
2010	Fast food (cod filet sandwich + cheese curds + med coke)	lunch
	Fast food (chicken sandwich + sm fries + sm coke)	
	Fast food (spicy chicken sandwich + med coke)	
2011	various (due to team lunches)	lunch
2012	various (due to team lunches)	lunch
2013	Fast food (filet-o-fish + sm fries + sm coke)	lunch
2014	Fast food (2 large xtra crispy breasts + cole slaw + med coke)	lunch
2015	Fast food (spicy chicken sandwich + med coke)	lunch

Below, is another snapshot analysis that I did that tracked what I ordered from the same health food store for lunch. It shows the same items I would order and for how many days at-a-time I would order them. This wasn't a concurrent thing; this was a consecutive thing in that I would last for 123 days ordering the same thing then move on to the next thing for 49 days… then the next thing for 44 days… and so-on.

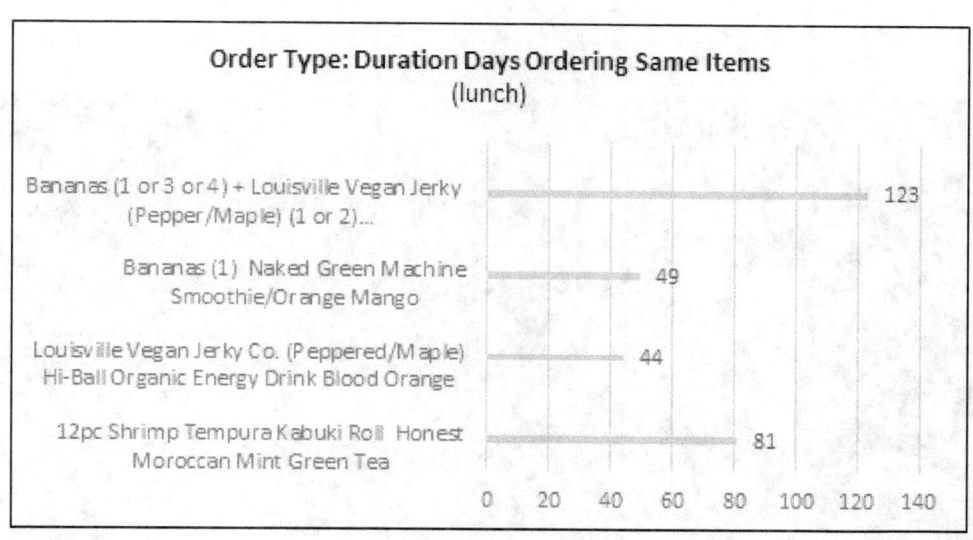

Coping Mechanisms

A coping mechanism involves making use of any calming technique or device (which can also include alcohol or other substances for some people---developing into bad habits, as a result, if gone unchecked). Stimming, for example, falls under this category (more on that, later).

The moment I get into a restaurant or bar or dance club, if there is a pen and a napkin or back of receipt or a tray, I will draw on it. I do it to calm myself down more than anything else, but various people have enjoyed the artwork (I've given many signed napkins to workers over the years). Below, are two photos that show how focused I can be while using this particular coping mechanism. It is ritual. It is helpful. It is also a bit odd.

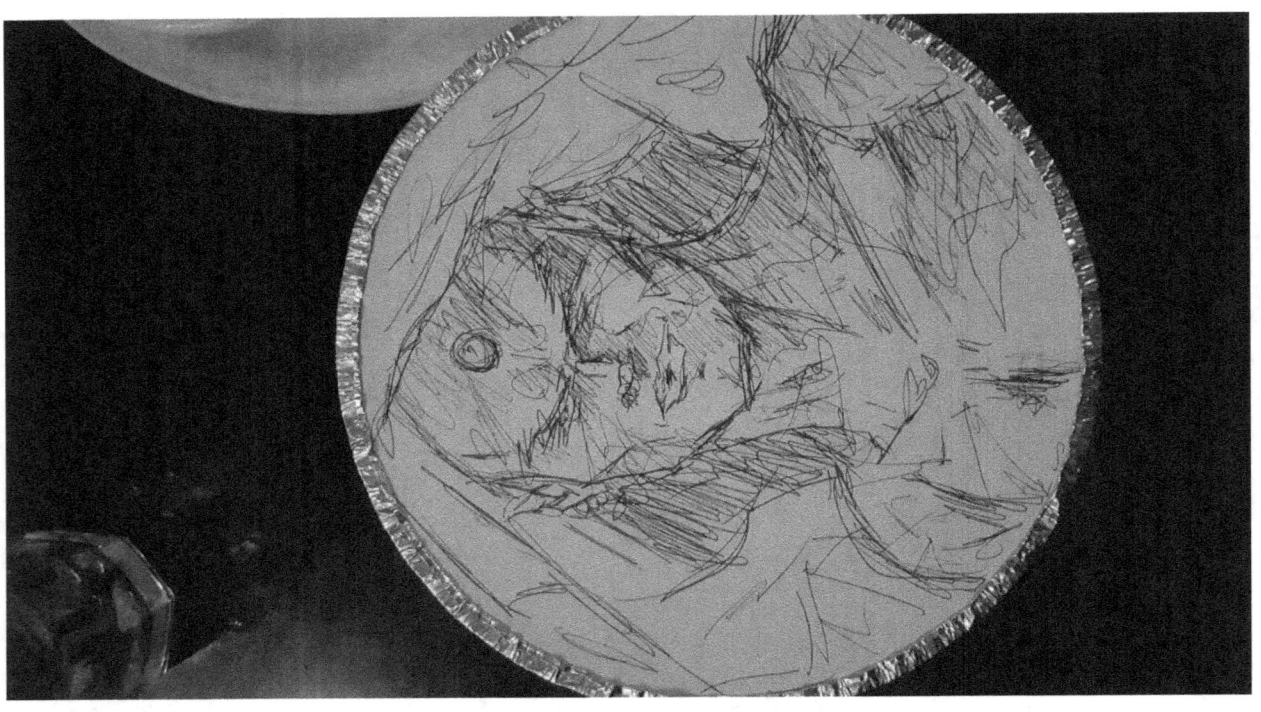

Figure 1 random drawing on a to-go container at a restaurant

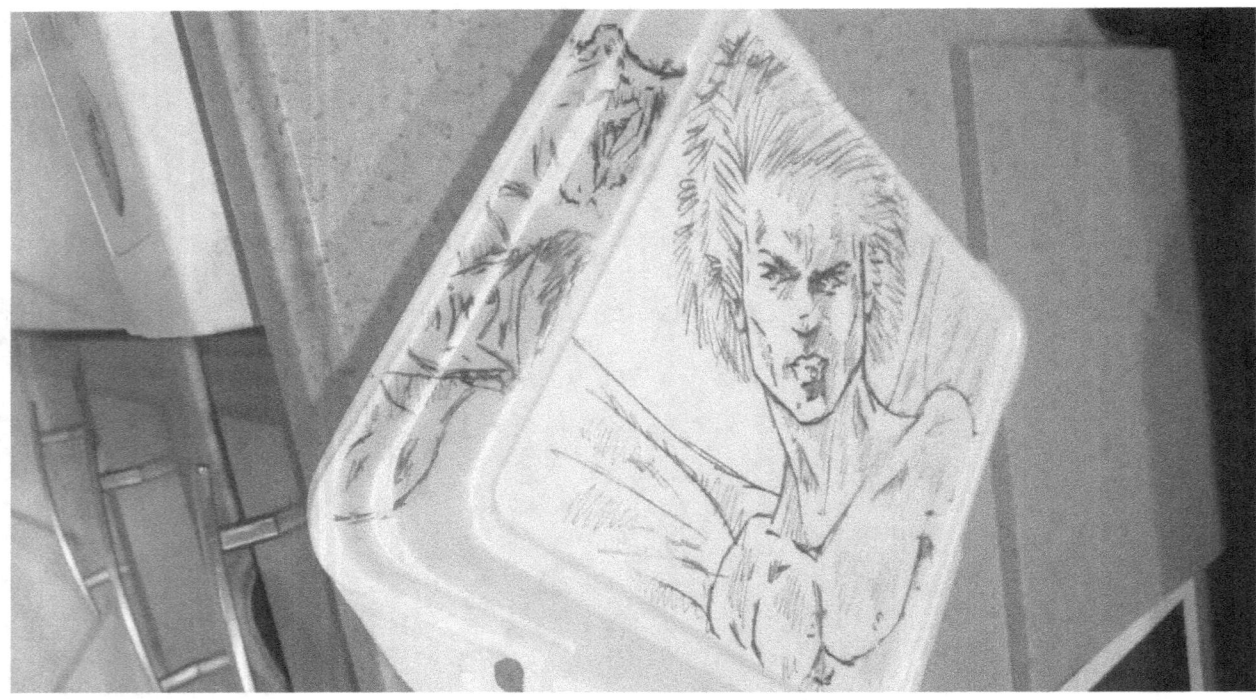

Figure 2 random drawing on a to-go container at a restaurant

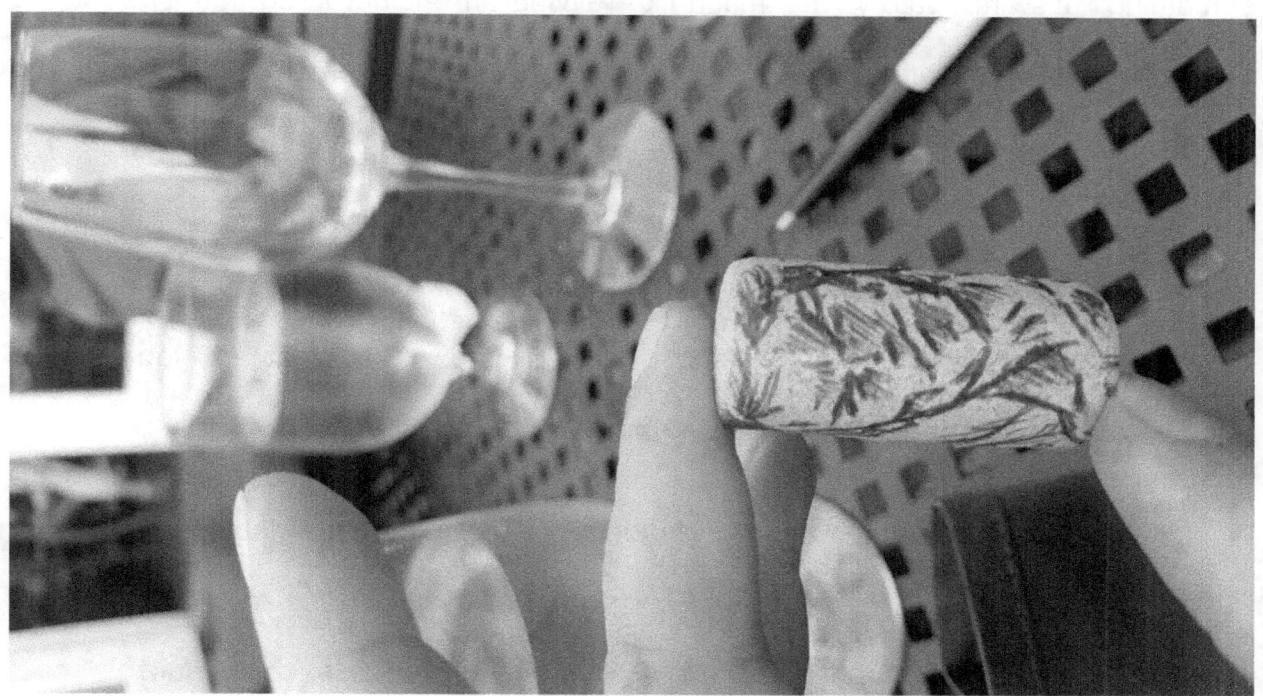

Figure 3 random drawing on a wine cork at a restaurant

One of my favourite things to do is to take a photo of each item I've drawn and post it on social media. In a way, it's an inside joke to myself. In another way, I'm just sharing my illustrations to the world.

At one point, I used to draw on the puke bags that airlines used to keep behind the seats. This was before it occurred to me to start bringing my drawing supplies with me on flights. I've given away numerous drawings to flight attendants (if they commented on them).

Stimming. Below, are snapshots of me finger tapping. I do this when I'm excited about something or nervous about something---mostly, when I'm excited about something. It's anticipatory. It's much like revving an engine up so that it's ready to take off. Self-stimulating motor movements are quite common in folks on The Spectrum. They vary as much as the person's personality. Some (especially seen in kids) rock back-and-forth or side-to-side; others flap their hands, spin around in circles, tap their foot, etc. I've done this since early childhood. Mom could tell when I was nervous about something because she would ask me: "ok. What are you nervous about? You're digging under your nails, again."

The following 3 photos are of me doing my "penguin flipper" tapping. I typically do this when I'm exited about something or revving myself up for something exciting about to happen. I've caught myself doing this during meetings, conversations about topics I'm actually interested in, before and while playing video games, and especially while listening to music (specific songs I love):

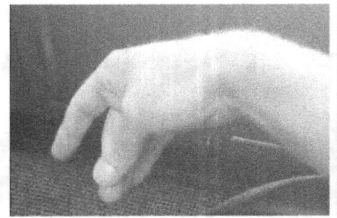 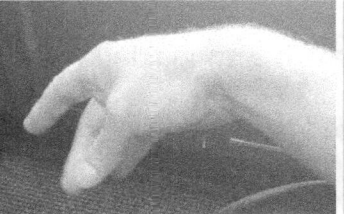 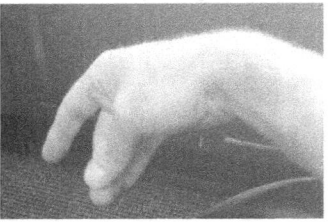

Below, is another snapshot of me finger tapping, rapidly. I'll do this as a favourite song is coming on the radio while driving; I'll do this when I'm trying to figure out an issue/researching something; I'll do this just as my favourite video game is about to start; I'll do this while in a movie theater just before the main movie starts. This is just another stimulatory example and something I do far more often than I was originally aware of. This is not like regular finger tapping that most people do to the beat of a song. This is usually a rapid-fire reaction that happens involuntarily and even in the absence of other sounds in the room.

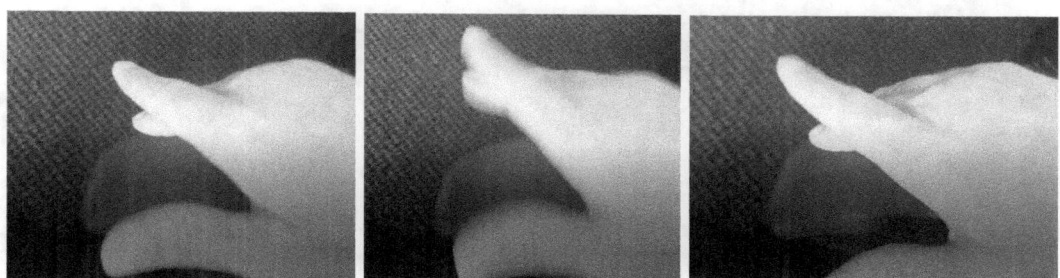

Below, is another snapshot of a stimming behaviour I do only when I'm nervous about something. This is a telltale sign that I'm extremely nervous about something that's about to happen. This, too, is anticipatory and involuntary. I dig under my nails. Each nail, one at-a-time.

I've learned this coping mechanism while dancing. Someone like me takes a long time to get used to a dance floor and the people already occupying it---and the lights, sounds, sensations that go with it. Once I've "found my groove," I can start to adapt to the beat of the music playing. I snap my fingers quite often (even when I'm not dancing), and it looks like I'm just snapping to the beat of the music, but I'm actually just stimming. The act keeps my mind focused on the calming, snapping sensation, and not on the unpredictable dance floor---which keeps the anxiety from building up.

Chapter Conclusion

It is an easy thing to confuse OCD (Obsessive-compulsive Disorder) with compulsiveness regarding autism since both rely upon repetition. One is unpleasant and restrictive while the other is desirable and often by choice---willingly repeating a thing because it is "safe" and predictable (known).

FORMAL DIAGNOSIS

Pre-diagnosis

In 2017, as an adult, I was formally diagnosed with Autism Spectrum Disorder (Level I) along with Psychological Factors Affecting Other Medical Conditions (the anxiety-induced muscle/skeletal pains during/after social interactions).

Having grown-up feeling different, not being able to interact socially the way others normally/naturally could, having experienced sensory issues, being stuck in routines, preferring a sense of sameness, experiencing consequences for not making regular adjustments, and having other side-effects from… something, I knew I needed to seek answers as I was gradually realizing something was at the root cause of it all.

During my teens, some people would see me drawing on a bench in the mall or at a restaurant or on an airplane or… and they would say "oh, you're so artistic!" My response: "no, I'm autistic not artistic." I was making a sort-of inside joke at myself because I suspected it back then. I had not yet mastered the art of tactful reply, and I took many things quite literally, so my bluntness was quite apparent.

As I've mentioned in previous books, Martial Arts had been a special interest of mine since 1988. I would get muscle pains at seemingly-random times that I couldn't explain. I would be short-of-breath, tire easily, break-out in heavy sweat, and basically look like I was dying after some sessions with training partners or while in classes. What I didn't realize until just over one year ago was the pain was a result of anxiety--- caused from training with other people (aka social interaction on a physical level). I had to replay the scenarios in my head from years ago and start documenting when it was occurring---what were the variables? I can't be convinced of anything until I see the data. I concluded that each time I came into close proximity with another person---there was prolonged physical contact (like wrestling), in just 5 minutes my body would start tensing-up, fatigue would kick-in, the sweating process would start… in short, it was an anxiety attack.

I described it as having sawdust filling-up inside my limbs. I remember my very last JiuJitsu class (it was only 1 hour) was my drawing-point. I was at a point only 30 minutes into the session where I could barely move, barely get off the mat.

See, I could still deal with everything else in my life, but I could not allow the muscle/skeletal (psychosomatic) pains to consume my life any longer. I was forced to drop-out of my Catch-as-Catch-Can Wrestling and Brazilian JiuJitsu training sessions because of it. Learning and retaining the techniques simply came naturally to me even after just a few drills, but I couldn't last long enough beyond 15 minutes in each class. It would take me exactly 3 days for my body to recover from the anxiety attacks. This was unacceptable.

At this time, I went to a movie theater to see The Imitation Game™. I had no idea what it was about, but my friend encouraged the rest of us to go see it with him. I did not know who Alan Turing was. There were several points during the movie that I began to cry because I saw some similarities between the character being portrayed and myself---not the savant-like brilliance of Turing but the bullying and conversation and quirks.

I started doing my own research on social disorders, ADHD, Asperger's Syndrome, Autism, etc.

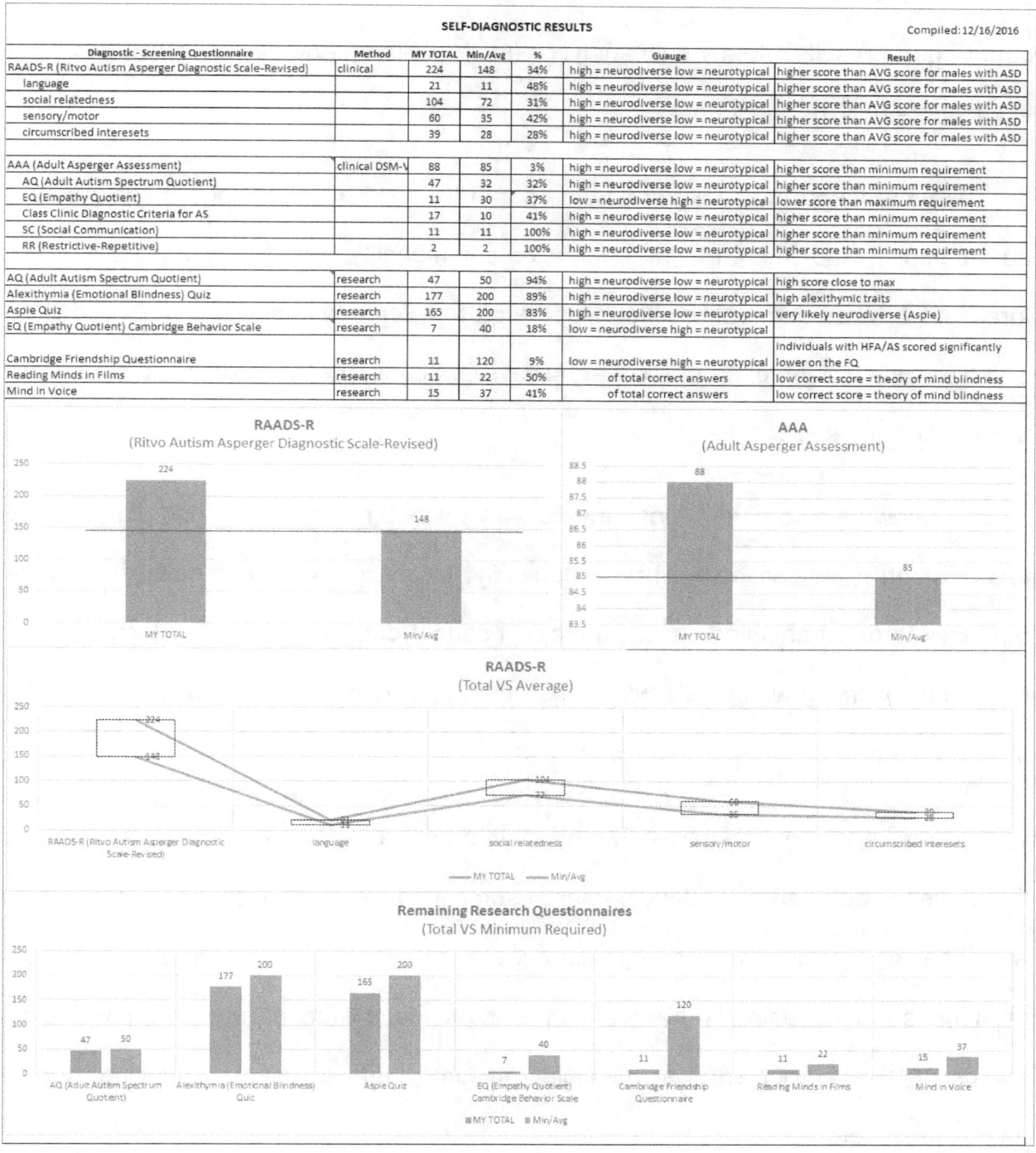

Thanks to the power of online shared knowledge, I came across several websites, newsgroups, and individual blogs by people who had already completed their own journeys and shared some of their experiences. Some even created their own tools to help others. I began taking as many online self-diagnosis tests I could, compiled the results into my own analytics (image above), and quickly concluded I was somewhere on The Spectrum.

Even though my background was not in the field of psychology, I knew how to pull, compile, and interpret data---look for commonality, remove inconsistency, and forecast the remaining results... look for the cross-reference in psychology-based texts. Self-diagnosis wasn't enough for me, however, because I require official confirmation, so I needed professional feedback.

I knew I was onto the root cause of why I was the way I was---and possibly how to work with it instead of against it (hopefully, to learn how to dull-down my natural tendency to resist anything attacking me). I sought-out a social worker, first, who had experience working with adults with Asperger's, and he was quite helpful in confirming my suspicions.

I spoke with my primary care physician during a routine physical and mentioned that I suspected I had a "social disorder of some kind" and also mentioned to her that I was seeing a social worker regarding t. We had already been discussing the mysterious muscle pains I'd been experiencing since childhood but could never find a source of it (ruled-out arthritis, muscular myopathy due to certain medicine, sports-related injury, etc.).

She referred me to a local neuropsychology testing facility, and the closing of my first journey was at-hand.

Below, is the actual timeline:

2016	Nov	Began self-diagnosis/research process
2016	Dec	Began seeing a social worker/counselor who also worked with people with Asperger's Syndrome in the past
2017	Jan	Referral from primary care physician to neuropsychology testing facility after mentioning a suspicion of a "social disorder of some kind." Submitted initial screening questionnaire.
2017	Mar	9th initial interview/consultation (1.5 hrs.) First test (CPT Continuous Performance Test) to rule out ADHD (15 min) 22nd primary interview (6 hrs.)
2017	Jun	16th formal testing process (6 hrs.) 20th testing cont'd/follow-up interview (2 hrs.)
2017	Jul	11th test results (1.5 hrs.)
2017	Aug	18th test results cont'd (1.5 hrs.) Official Diagnosis: Autism Spectrum Disorder Level 1 F84.0 (2.5 hrs.) Comorbid Diagnosis: Psychological Factors Affecting Other Medical Conditions F54 General Intellectual Ability Above Average Intelligence Self-Diagnosis/Research Total Time: 7 months (concurrent) Social Worker/Counselor Total Time: 4 hours (1 hr. sessions) Formal Diagnosis Total Time: 20.5 hours

Diagnosis

This was the most important series of steps I could have ever taken, and I am quite content and thankful for having done so. My neuropsychologist was experienced, personable, and knowledgeable. I couldn't have asked for a better person to help me during the diagnosis process, and I learned MUCH from him.

I'm analytical by nature, so I had to understand each test, how it broke things down, compile everything into my own analytics and interpret the results visually so that I could better understand them. My neuropsychologist knew this about me, so he would explain what I was in for. It was not easy for him because I supplied HUNDREDS of pages of examples and compiled a historical document (from infancy through current), so there was undoubtedly too much information supplied. Also, of note: adults on The Spectrum are very difficult to diagnose, formally, because we learn coping mechanisms and adaptive techniques to mostly compensate for our difficulties. Some of us learn to mask ourselves and hide inside a sort-of mental "cave." Some of us didn't make it into adulthood because the support mechanisms were not available at the time, and the pressure/depression/etc. were simply too much.

Most people think of psychological examinations as negative things. They think there is a "crazy" associated with them. They think if they simply avoid it altogether, they will never have to come face-to-face with the mental challenges EACH of us face on a CONSTANT basis. It isn't just Autism Spectrum Disorder… I would challenge someone to NOT be on a spectrum of some kind or to not have a mental disorder or emotional imbalance or… I don't believe such a person exists.

The neuropsychological examination is slightly different from a standard psychological examination. A neuropsychological exam focuses on a process-of-elimination method (called differential diagnosis) to help isolate very specific disorders and to better tailor treatment or coping techniques to better live with them. I was quite fortunate that the facility I was tested at doesn't prescribe meds as a first resort but has a culture of behaviour modification instead. I'm not a med fan, personally, but meds are necessary for those extreme cases.

The CPT (Continuous Performance Test) was the only computer-based test I took. Everything else was pencil and paper and observation. I went into the entire process suspecting it would take more than one visit, a great deal of patience, concentration, and complete honesty (self-honesty). As I started the test, my neuropsychologist was quickly explaining the rules to me, and I simply could not see the screen while he was talking---I could only "see" what he was explaining to me, so I was already missing some of the visual cues (this goes back to hyperfocus).

The CPT took about 15 minutes, but it felt more like 5 to me. It was like playing a video game, and I was having fun enduring the challenge. The goal was to press the keyboard spacebar key each time there was a specific letter that flashed on the screen. The duration before, during, and after would vary, so I couldn't get away with counting the times/pacing. Even though I knew the goal was to be accurate and fast, I was simply fast (my reaction time was in the "very superior" result) and quite inaccurate. I clicked far more often on the wrong letters than I should have. This test is one that helps differentiate ADHD because it shows concentration impairments (distraction/ impatience/ impulse). I was simply impulsive.

Because I was entrenched into this entire process, having researched as much as I already had---coupled with my hyperfocus---the timeframe did not seem long to me. Some testing dates lasted several hours (see the timeline above), but they would pass like mere minutes to me.

Below, are groupings of the tests and how they were classified:

Neuropsychological Evaluation

category	test	classification
Intellectual Functioning	WAIS-IV Full-Scale IQ (FSIQ)	Average
	WAIS-IV Verbal Comprehension Index (VCI)	Superior
	WAIS-IV Perceptual Reasoning Index (PRI)	High Average
	WAIS-IV Working Memory Index (WMI)	Average
	WAIS-IV Processing Speed Index (PSI)	Impaired
	North American Adult Reading Test (NAART)	Average
Language & Overlearned Info	WAIS-IV Information	Superior
	WAIS-IV Vocabulary	High Average
Verbal Reasoning & Judgment	WAIS-IV Similarities	Average
Academic Skills	WAIS-IV Arithmetic	Average
Non-Verbal Perception & Reasoning	WAIS-IV Matrix Reasoning	Superior
	WAIS-IV Visual Puzzles	Superior
Visuospatial Construction & Praxis	WAIS-IV Block Design	High Average
	Rey-O Copy	Average

Neuropsychological Evaluation

category	test	classification
Attention & Concentration	Trails A	Impaired
	WAIS-IV Digits Forward	Borderline
	NAB-N&L A efficiency (sustained attention)	Impaired
	Continuous Performance Test - omission errors	Average
	Continuous Performance Test - variability	Impaired
Tracking & Processing Speed	WAIS-IV Symbol Search	Impaired
	WAIS-IV Coding	Borderline
	NAB-N&L A speed (sustained attention)	Impaired
	Trails A (simple scanning and tracking)	Impaired
Executive Functioning	Stroop	Impaired
	Trails B (simultaneous double tracking)	Low Average
	NAB - N&L D efficiency (complex divided attention)	Impaired
	Continuous Performance Test - commission errors	Average
	Continuous Performance Test - perseverative errors	Average

Neuropsychological Evaluation

category	test	classification
Working Memory	WAIS-IV Digits Backward	Low Average
	WAIS-IV Digit Span Sequencing	Low Average
	WAIS-IV Arithmetic	High Average
	NAB - N&L B (selective attention)	Low Average
	NAB - N&L C (selective attention)	Low Average
Verbal Immediate Memory	NAB - Story Learning - Immediate Recall	High Average
Verbal Short-Term Memory	NAB Story Learning - Delayed Recall	High Average
Verbal Memory, Learning	NAB List Learning A - Immediate Recall	Low Average
	NAB List Learning A - Short Delay Recall	Average
	NAB List Learning - Long Delay Recall	Average
	Rey-O Immediate Recall	Borderline
Visual Short-Term Memory	Rey-O Delayed Recall	Low Average
Visual Memory, Learning	Rey-O Recognition	Low Average

At first glance, anyone receiving test results like above might panic and/or feel quite proud. It isn't until you break down each test and what it's gauging that you realize a low average or a superior or... is really reflecting specific mental areas and not the overall mental status of a person. These results help the diagnostician gather a better understanding for a possible diagnosis (or non-diagnosis). The tests also help flag overall mental impairment (damage, deficiency [such as intellectual disability] or degradation [such as dementia]).

You may notice there are some extremes in my test results. This is quite common for folks who are on The Spectrum because we have a polarized imbalance in overall mental focus/ prioritization/ function. We have really high points and really low points, and everything else is in-between. "Normal" people who would go through these tests would score slightly differently in several categories (typically in the average score result with little-to-no extreme results).

Those of us on The Spectrum are often weak in mental perception because we require more concrete objects to focus on. Our processing speed is often impaired. We can figure things out (in my case, patterns) when given the topic, but it will take us longer than most other people.

I absolutely struggled through most of the verbal portions because I need to SEE things in order to fully comprehend them. I knew the results in this area were going to be poor---and they were. This is simply data that helps explain why I have to write things down when I'm on the phone (and why I hate talking on the phone... period). This explains the numerous challenges I experience during a simple conversation because I have to replay the experience over-and-over in my head afterwards. It explains why there is a significant delay in my own emotional reciprocity (I have to think about what was said before I can get angry or happy or remain unemotional about it).

The verbal word problems were immensely challenging for me because I didn't have two very important compensatory tools: 1) pencil/paper or 2) Microsoft Excel. When I was growing up, I absolutely struggled through math of any kind---with the exception of applied physics and geometry (one has an actual logic behind the formulae and the other is purely visual and adheres to my lifelong special interest in shapes). It wasn't until I mastered Excel that I was able to compensate because I understood the tables and rows---taking a math problem out of its original context and putting it in a context I could better understand. Essentially, I have to rely HEAVILY on technical tools.

My strengths, not surprising to me, were in the visuals. I love patterns and see patterns in everything I notice. When we reached the puzzles section, I was so excited about getting into them that I was stimming (finger tapping like I normally do when I hear a song I love or... pretty much anything I love) heavily.

The brain is like a computer; a computer is like the brain. In the world of psychology, there are certain terms that are used frequently during the diagnosis stage for a patient to better understand how test results and treatment options apply. I had difficulty visualizing what "working memory" and "rote memory" and "processing speed" versus reaction time looked like. The only way I could truly comprehend these variables was to compare them to something I could visualize---a computer. Again, most folks on The Spectrum think in terms of visuals or pictures.

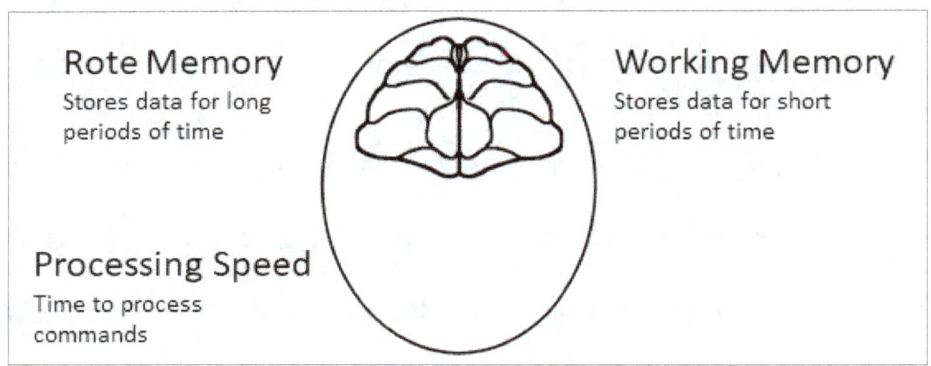

- Rote Memory – the brain's capacity to store items for long periods of time.

- Working Memory – the brain's capacity to store items for immediate recall (short periods of time).

- Processing Speed – the speed in which the brain receives and interprets information. The faster the processing speed, the faster the brain can do something with the information it just received. This is where the terms "fast acting" and "quick thinking" come into play.

Comparing the brain to a computer, a hard drive would equate to rote memory in that it stores data for long periods of time. RAM (random access memory) stores data for short periods of time and is responsible for immediate recall. A computer's processor is responsible for processing commands, and the higher its capacity, the faster its processing speed will be. If a computer's hard drive is high capacity, it can store large amounts of data. If a computer's RAM is low capacity, it can only store small amounts of data for shorter periods of time. If a computer's processor is low capacity, it's processing speed will be quite slow. Small RAM and a slow processor equate to a slow running computer. A human being on The Spectrum is much the same in this comparison.

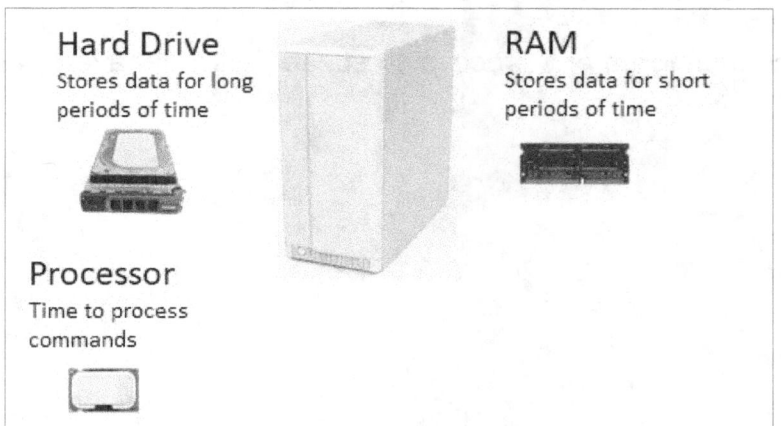

In my case, my "hard drive" (or rote memory) is excellent. I can retain/recall long term memory in detail (primarily visual but conversations tend to hold quite well here, as well – mainly due to my nature of replaying conversations over-and-over). My "RAM" (or working memory) is quite poor---especially in regards to audible situations where I have to write most things that I hear down on paper so that I can see them in order to comprehend and retain them. There is a difference between processing speed and reaction time. In my case, I have "very superior" reaction time but my processing speed is impaired. What this means for me is that it takes me more time to digest what is being told to me (if I hadn't already experienced it before, mind you) or shown to me. I require more time to think about things and interpret them. I have to make flowcharts or plug data into a spreadsheet and reinterpret results into something I can visualize---then make a decision as a result. Essentially, this means I have to over-analyze certain things in order to make a decision.

ADHD (Attention Deficit Hyperactivity Disorder) is a required differential diagnostic because it is quite common and has overlapping traits with other neurodevelopmental disorders. In fact, it's quite common for people on The Spectrum to have a comorbid diagnosis of ADHD. In my case, I was borderline enough that it was ruled-out as the primary contributor to any processing speed deficits I have. Below, are the test results:

	score	percentile	range	result
Adult Attention Deficit Disorders Evaluation Scale				
inattentive subscale	9	24th	Low average	infrequent symptoms of being distracted by external stimuli, having difficulty with activities requiring sustained listening, failing to pay attention to important sounds, difficulty concentrating when reading or following a conversation, failing to independently complete chores, failing to remain on task to prepare to work assignments, difficulty organizing tasks, difficulty getting started on a task, difficulty managing time at work, difficulty managing paperwork on the job, difficulty paying attention in conversation with fellow employees, failing to complete work assignments during work time, and failing to perform up to his potential at work.
hyperactive-impulsive subscale	9	24th	Low average	infrequent symptoms of interrupting others, impulsively reacting to situations without thinking, initiating responses before receiving directions or reading instructions, moving about while seated, having difficulty remaining seated for extended periods, feeling subjectively restless, handling objects such as pens or pencils excessively, moving about unnecessarily, making excessive noise, talking at inappropriate times, engaging in inappropriate behaviors while seated, interrupting others, and blurting out responses at work.

Note: percentile rank is determined against a percentage of test takers. The higher the percentage equals the higher on the ranking scale you may be. The lower the percentage equals the lower on the ranking scale you may be. It isn't quite like getting answers right or wrong on a quiz, but, more so, how your test results compare to others who have taken the same test.

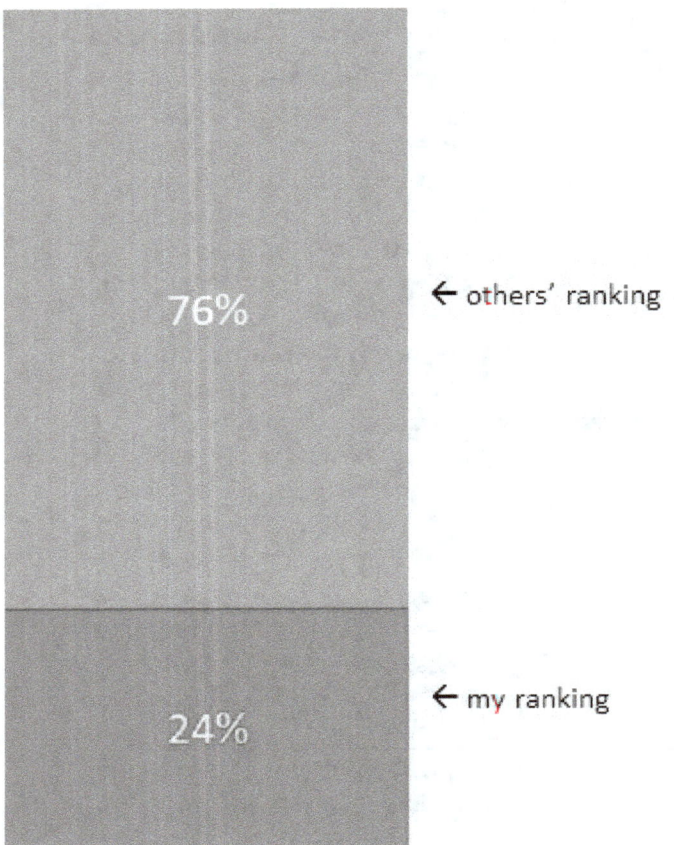

In my case, I scored somewhat low, overall, regarding the AADDES, compared to others who have taken it. This, along with CPT and other test subscales and the fact I've been the way I am since infancy/early childhood, helped differentiate (rule-out) ADHD as a primary condition.

There were enough overlaps in symptoms to not entirely rule-out the possibility of comorbid ADHD, but the autistic traits explain these overlaps more accurately than simple attention issues.

Even though Asperger's Syndrome no longer exists as its own diagnosis (as of 2013), it can still be used as part of the overall Autism Spectrum Disorder testing process. My particular portion was Q&A interview and observation-based:

		Asperger Syndrome Diagnostic Scale		
	score	percentile	range	result
asperger syndrome quotient subscale	105	n/a	n/a	likely
language subscale	13	84th	High Average	overly formal manner, talks excessively about limited area of interest, uses words or phrases repetitively, demonstrates difficulty understanding subtlety, sarcasm, interpret conversations literally, problems comprehending metaphors and idioms, difficulty initiating conversations
social subscale				does NOT exhibit peculiar voice characteristics
social subscale	8	25th	Low Average	difficulty relating to others, shows limited interest in other people, preferred to be in company of adults rather than peers, limited interest in what others say, difficulty understanding other's feelings, does not understand rules governing social behavior, limited ability to comprehend social cues
social subscale				does not use a limited number of gestures, does not avoid eye contact, does have the capacity to make friends, does not exhibit inappropriate facial expressions, able to respect others' space

		Asperger Syndrome Diagnostic Scale		
	score	percentile	range	result
maladaptive subscale	9	37th	Average	fails to change behavior to match environment, engages in inappropriate behavior related to obsessive or favorite interest, does exhibit strong reactions to changes in routine, does engage in repeated obsessive and/or ritualistic behavior, loses temper, does attempt to impose narrow interests, routines or structures on others
				does NOT demonstrate antisocial behavior, does not panic when unscheduled events occur, does not appear depressed, does not display immature behaviors, does not feel overwhelmed or bewildered in demanding situations

		Asperger Syndrome Diagnostic Scale		
	score	percentile	range	result
cognitive area subscale	13	84th	High Average	displays superior ability in a restricted area of interest, extreme interest in a narrow subject, functions best when engaged in familiar tasks, does have excellent rote memory, does learn best when pictures or written words are present, does have ABOVE AVERAGE intelligence, aware he is different from others, oversensitive to criticism, lacks common sense
sensorimotor functioning	13	84th	High Average	does NOT lack organizational skills demonstrates unusual reactions to loud, unexpected noises, does stiffen or pull away when hugged, is hypersensitive to smells, does show preference for certain fabrics, does have restricted diet consisting of the same foods cooked/presented the same way
				does NOT exhibit difficulty with fine motor skills or appear clumsy/uncoordinated

The Wechsler Adult Intelligence Scale (WAIS) test is a popular tool that is used by many schools, psychologists and other professionals to assist in the interpretation of intelligence [3]. The tests were intensely involved with some portions being quite fun and others being quite challenging. In fact, the majority of my entire diagnostics timeframe was taken-up by the WAIS.

There is a misconception that a person takes an IQ Test in order to see where he/she rates in terms of intelligence. We've all heard the phrase "I have a high IQ." The internet is peppered with IQ tests. Unless a person undergoes a full neuropsychological examination, those reported "IQ tests" are absolute rubbish and quite meaningless. There is far more to assessing intelligence than a simple test. I was taken-back by this, and it was refreshing to me that my educational attainments also factored-in. I actually expected to see a lower score in my results.

WAIS-IV Results			
WAIS-IV	score	result	Description
FSIQ	106	average	full scale overall cognitive abilities
VCI	108	average	verbal comprehension
PRI	115	high average	perceptual reasoning
WMI	100	average	working memory
PSI	89	low average	processing speed

General Intelligence Ability Level			
	score	result	description
NAART	111		performance on measures insensitive to injury mechanisms
GI		above average	general intelligence ability level based upon the highest scores from the testing profile, past academic achievement

In regards to the North American Adult Reading Test (NAART), it is a test that measures verbal intelligence but also helps determine if there is any potential brain trauma that may influence intellect to the negative (such as dementia).

The final grouping of it all is called General Intelligence. This couples past academic achievements with the WAIS test results.

I was pleased to see the "above average intelligence" result and was somewhat surprised. I never considered myself unintelligent, but I knew I was concentrated in my thought processes, and there are certain areas that I forever struggled with outside my "safe zones." I knew I had specialized areas I was intelligent in, but I knew there were others that would bring any scoring method down. The funny part (to me) is I didn't realize I was having my overall intelligence tested at the time. I simply "rolled with it" from one test to the next until completion.

The final summary to the entire diagnosis process was one of the first questionnaires I completed (over 400 questions in total). This was called the Millon Clinical Multiaxal Inventory (MCM-III). I could tell by the phrasing of the questions that this was a slightly dated compilation (from the 1980s, to be exact). I figured, however, that the more honest my answers were the more honest/accurate the results would be. This was the most "psychological" result finding out of all of the tests in that it attempted to break down a psychological profile of the test subject. Essentially, the elevated personality results from the MCMI-III pointed towards the social impairment effects of ASD and helped support the psychosomatic side-effects I'd been experiencing.

Official Diagnosis Results:

- Autism Spectrum Disorder Level I Without Accompanying Intellectual or Language Impairment (F84.0)

- Psychological Factors Affecting Other Medical Conditions (F54)

F84.0 and F54 are official diagnostic codes found in the International Statistical Classification of Diseases and Related Health Problems (ICD-10). In the United States (and some other countries), there is the aforementioned DSM-V and the ICD-10. In the States, diagnostics facilities use the DSM for determining psychological evaluation categories and sub-categories and, essentially, use it as the governing body. The facilities use the ICD-10 for the actual medical coding. As of this writing, these two versions are the most current (ICD version 10 and DSM version 5).

What was my reaction?

It was not surprise. It was relief. It was... affirmation.

Treatment and Cognitive-Behavioral Options were the next step. This part I was both ready and not ready for. I had an official explanation for the muscle pains I'd been experiencing. I knew it wasn't due to some other health reason. Great. Now what? How do I overcome everything else that actually helped me get to this point in my life? Well, it was logic and analytics that helped me get started; it would be logic and analytics to help me finish it. The first step: list each item that needs to be worked-on. The second step: detail each item and note if it needs to be eliminated or worked with instead of against. The third step: list and detail how to do it all.

For example, the way to better taper my hyperfocus is to bring myself DOWN when I'm in that state so that time does not go by so fast, and I end up missing other opportunities. When I'm bored (which is rare), I need to find activities that help me stay within "my groove" or my threshold of contentment.

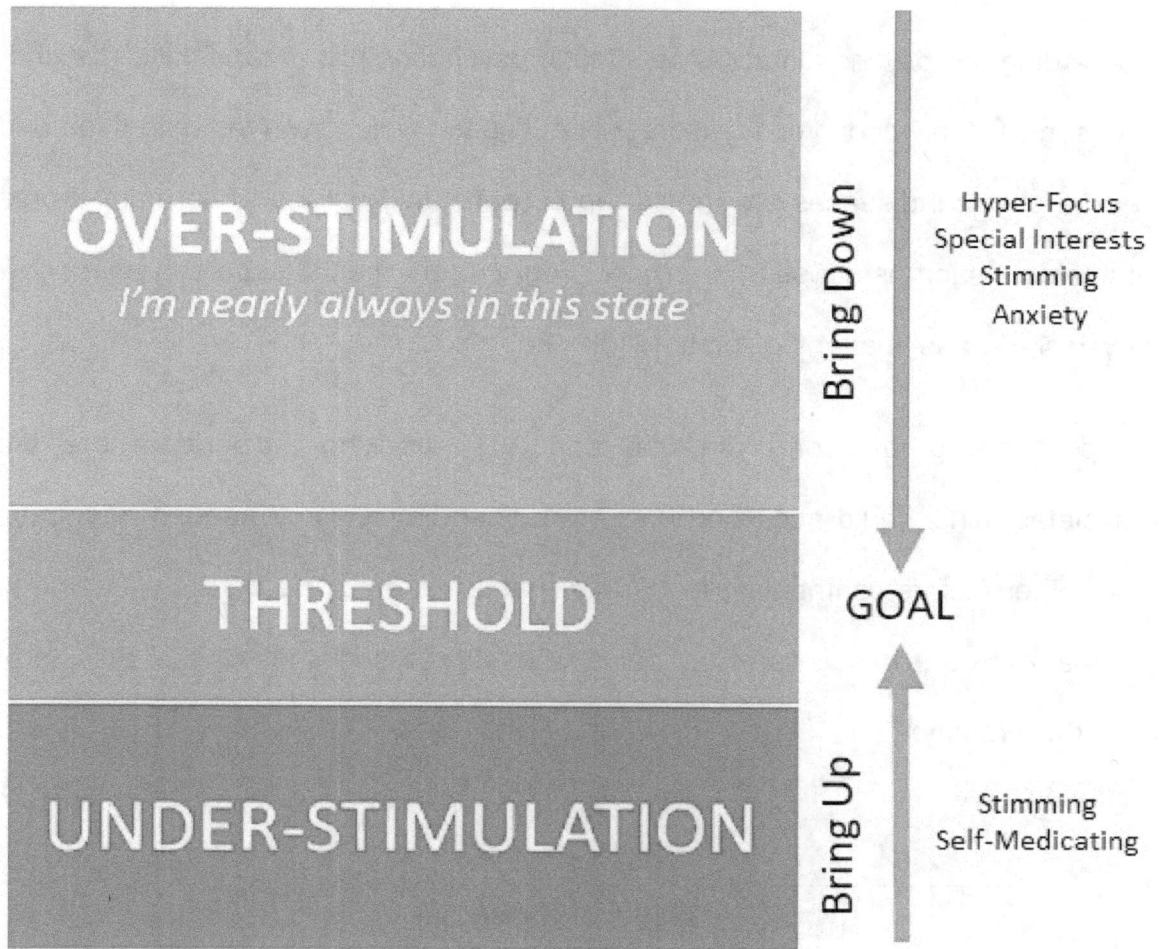

The other items, I've been teaching myself all along, anyway. I've taken numerous social and communication courses in college (with a special course in interpersonal communication that focused on body language). Something like this will never come second nature, but I can, at least, pause long enough to recall what I've learned and apply it to a situation.

There are aspects to this disorder that are useful and other aspects that are not harmful at all, so there's no point in doing anything about them.

Comorbid Diagnosis

Regarding the psychosomatic side-effects, psychosomatic means mind (psyche) and body (soma). A psychosomatic disorder is a disease which involves both mind and body. Some physical diseases are thought to be particularly prone to be made worse by mental factors such as stress and anxiety. Your current mental state can affect how bad a physical disease is at any given time [4].

I spent the greater part of 2016 and 2017 tracking incidents where the muscle/skeletal pains would occur, prior to my formal diagnosis. I needed to know if there were other factors contributing to it. After gathering empirical data, I was able to conclude that 42% of the source of my pains were due to social interaction outside of my normal daily routine.

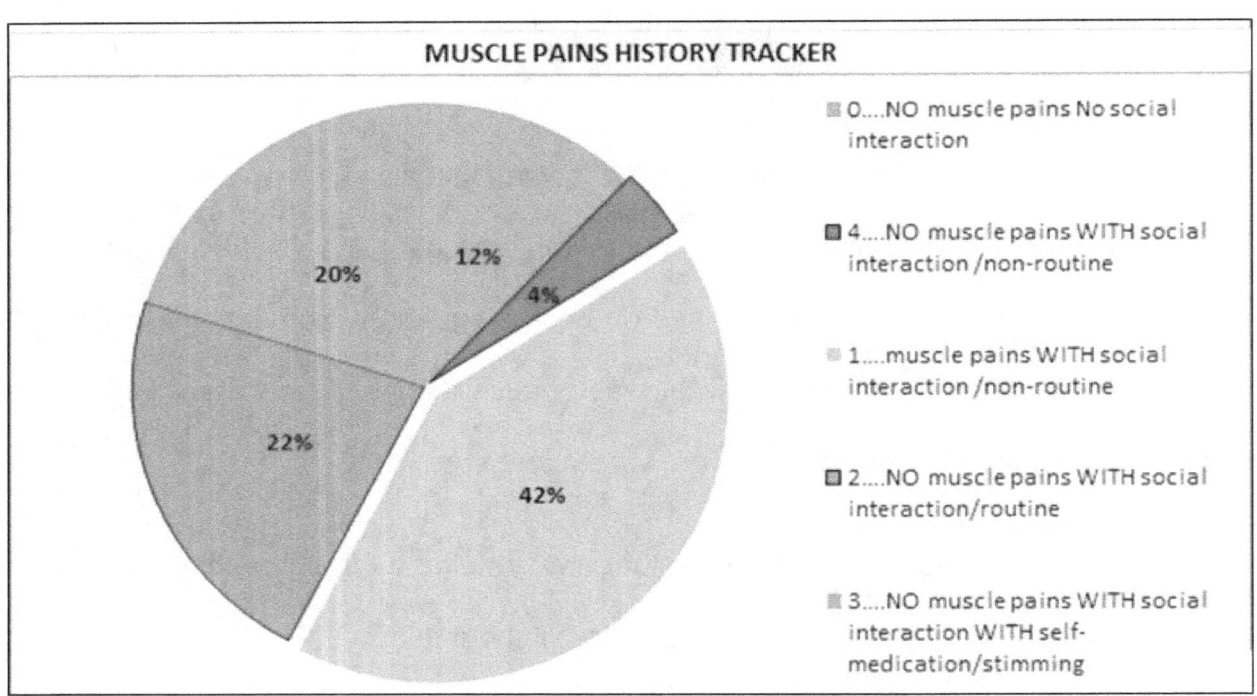

This is the primary reason I received a comorbid diagnosis of Psychological Factors Affecting Other Medical Conditions. It didn't qualify for a social anxiety disorder diagnosis because the autism is the source of the 2nd disorder. One is created from the other, in my case.

I also tracked the number of times I felt fatigue (not just a random sense of being tired, but extreme fatigue where I had to take 1 or more naps that lasted longer than 30 minutes) as a result of social interaction or some other source. I discovered over 75% of my fatigue or oversleep was after social interactions. Essentially, social interaction is incredibly draining to someone like me, whether I enjoy it or not. Not only does it cause me pain, it drains me.

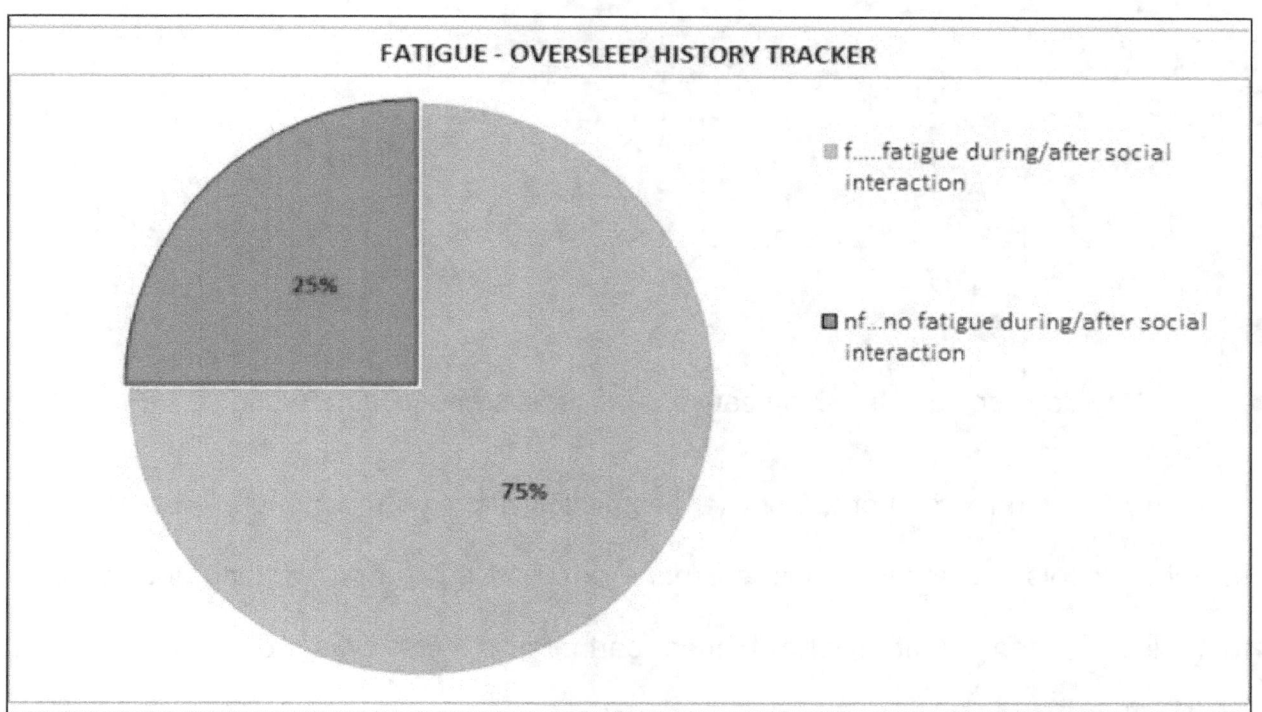

I was quite dialed-down with my analysis. I wanted to know what I was dealing with/what had been plaguing me since early childhood. I wanted to track the duration, group size, crowd size, whether I was driving or not, coping mechanisms, stimming method, pain location and intensity, and additional comments. My results were conclusive. Below, is a snapshot from one month of the type of data and classifications I was capturing:

APRIL Snapshot - Social Interaction - Pain and Coping Details

Date	Day	location	social type	group size (small (1 to 5) med (5 to 9) lrg (over 9))	crowd size (small (5 to 15) med (15 to 25) lrg (over 25))	soc mts	driving?	coping mechanism	coping amount (small (1 to 5) med (5 to 9) lrg (over 9))	stimming type	muscle pain?	pain location	pain intensity (light (ache) med (sharp) heavy (intense))	pain duration (short (under 1 hr) mod (1 to 3 hrs) long (over 3 hrs))	comments
4/1	Sat	home	domestic	small	none	0.00	no	none	none	none	no	none	none	none	
4/2	Sun	restaurant	social	small	large	120.00	no	alcohol	small	none	no	none	none	none	
4/3	Mon	restaurant	social	medium	medium	120.00	no	alcohol	small	none	no	none	none	none	
4/4	Tue	unknown	social	unknown	unknown	0.00	unknown	unknown	unknown	unknown	yes	unknown	unknown	unknown	
4/5	Wed	restaurant	social	medium	medium	120.00	no	alcohol	small	none	no	none	none	none	
4/6	Thu	work	work	small	small	0.00	yes	music	large	none	no	none	none	none	
4/7	Fri	home	domestic	small	small	0.00	no	none	none	none	none	none	none	none	
4/8	Sat	convention	social	small	large	540.00	yes	costume/alcohol	small	none	no	none	none	none	in costume entire time
4/9	Sun	restaurant	social	small	medium	90.00	no	stimming/alcohol	small	drawing	no	none	none	none	
4/10	Mon	work	work	small	small	60.00	yes	none	none	none	yes	right front hip	light	short	meeting with AT&T
4/11	Tue	restaurant	social	small	medium	90.00	no	alcohol	small	none	no	none	none	none	
4/12	Wed	work/home	work/solo	small	small	0.00	yes	music	large	none	no	none	none	none	
4/13	Thu	work/home/the	solo	none	medium	120.00	no	movie	small	finger tapping	no	none	none	none	Rifftrax Samurai Cop
4/14	Fri	restaurant/club	social	small	large	180.00	no	alcohol	small	none	yes	left hamstring	medium	short	went away after coping
4/15	Sat	restaurant/club	social	medium	medium/large	360.00	no	alcohol	small	none	yes	right hip	heavy	long	
4/16	Sun	restaurant	social	small	medium	90.00	no	none	none	none	no	none	none	none	
4/17	Mon	work/home	work/solo	none	small	0.00	yes	music	large	none	no	none	none	none	
4/18	Tue	restaurant	social	small	medium	0.00	no	alcohol	small	none	yes	right hip/hams	medium	short	went away after coping
4/19	Wed	work	work	small	small	30.00	yes	none	none	none	yes	left hip	light	short	conference call Fedline
4/19	Wed	dept stores/hom	shopping/solo	none	large	120.00	yes	none	none	none	yes	left shoulder	medium	short	
4/20	Thu	hospital/work/h	appt	small	small	60.00	yes	stimming	small	finger tapping	no	none	none	none	
4/21	Fri	work/home	work/solo	none	small	0.00	yes	music	large	none	no	none	none	none	
4/22	Sat	home	solo	none	none	720.00	no	music	large	none	no	none	none	none	working on costume
4/23	Sun	dept stores	shopping	small	large	180.00	yes	none	none	none	yes	right hip/hams	heavy	long	continued into Monday went away after getting Home from Work (Mon)
4/24	Mon	work	work/solo	none	small	0.00	yes	music	large	none	yes	right hip/hams	heavy	long	residual from yesterday - went away once Home
4/25	Tue	work/home	work/solo	none	small	0.00	yes	music	large	none	no	none	none	none	
4/26	Wed	work/home	work/domestic	small	small	0.00	yes	music	medium	none	no	none	none	none	
4/27	Thu	work/home	work/domestic	small	small	0.00	yes	music	medium	none	no	none	none	none	
4/28	Fri	work/home	work/domestic	small	small	0.00	yes	music	medium	none	no	none	none	none	
4/29	Sat	restaurant	social	medium	medium	90.00	no	stimming/alcohol	small	drawing	no	none	none	none	
4/29	Sat	club	social	small	large	60.00	no	stimming/alcohol	small	finger tapping	yes	rear hips	light	short	went away after getting Home
4/30	Sun	park	social	small	large	60.00	no	none	none	none	no	none	none	none	

Why does social interaction cause such drastic effects on the body?

When you read all of the challenges an autistic mind must endure, coupled with social protocols and expectations, someone on The Spectrum is working double, if not triple, just to keep up with his/her friends, partners, and co-workers on a near-constant basis. It's no wonder it takes a toll on the body.

Our bodies were not designed by nature to withstand constant punishment (in this case, constant stress) without giving way... somewhere. The manifestations can be pain in the left hip, pain in the right shoulder, pain in a knee... debilitatingly-intense pain wherever the body can choose to focus all of that negative energy.

Dealing with threshold is an easier task than dealing with minimizing psychosomatic effects of socializing. To my surprise, I was able to minimize it in a far shorter period of time than I anticipated. I researched other meditation techniques beyond controlled breathing methods (which are helpful, mind you). I learned how to meditate through movement using martial arts and studying Taoist energy flow concepts (similar to Tai Chi and Baqua). I discovered that the slowed movements of my Gung Fu background actually worked in a like manner.

The most important technique I learned, however, was to simply STOP thinking about it---before and during a social engagement of any kind, I learned how to not think about any of it. It was that simple. I saw and noted a significant drop in psychosomatic pain. It will never truly go away because it's a part of me, but I can work WITH it instead of AGAINST it, and the best way is to not feed the anxiety with any more mental fuel than it already has. I now go into social situations and don't think about the other people in them... I don't think about what they may be thinking about me... I don't think about the sensory overloads... I've learned how to numb myself.

Chapter Conclusion

Confirmation and affirmation are interesting concepts, especially when they are delved-out by other entities (or a 3rd party institution). At times, it isn't enough to

KNOW you have or are a thing---you need someone else to confirm it. There is a sense of helplessness regarding this, but I have no regrets having undergone the entire process and am better for it. I can't recommend a formal diagnosis (where possible) enough.

HOW I PERCEIVE THE WORLD

This particular chapter simply focuses on how the autistic brain---my particular brain---perceives The World around it. In my case, I see geometric shapes in all things at all times (except for human faces). When I scan a room or a landscape or the outside of a building, I see the shapes FIRST and the content SECOND. Rarely is the subject matter relevant to me. I can be at a party or in a restaurant or on a cruise ship… or in a restroom---and, if the right shape catches my eye, I'm going to do whatever I can to capture it (in an illustration or a photograph).

This is not a photography book, however, although it may look like one. In fact, I'm not a photographer. I've never taken photography classes, but these are my own photographs.

This chapter captures how I see things. If it looks aesthetically pleasing, so be it. In fact, most things are aesthetically pleasing to me. You'll see a LOT of everyday objects that most people take for granted. It will become quite apparent that there are patterns throughout this book. When I was a child, I stared at walls and picture frames and ornaments and Christmas lights and car dashes… part of it was me trying to comprehend the item's purpose at the time… the rest of it was me appreciating and trying to absorb the beauty of the angles, shapes, intersections, and dimensions.

For the most part, colour is irrelevant to me. A black-and-white sunset is every bit as beautiful and terrifying as one in colour.

One thing you may notice (I did after it was pointed-out to me because I had no idea I was doing this the entire time) is that, if there is a human subject in the photograph, it was by accident. Human beings simply don't interest me nearly as much as the patterns on a coffee shop floor or the shadows cast by a half-full glass sitting on a copper tabletop. That's part of why I am what I am.

One more thing you may notice is the extreme ZOOM of things. I like to describe it as looking at everything through a telescope (or microscope). Even my illustrations are of close-up sections and partial faces or half torsos simply because I find the entirety of a thing to be uninteresting as opposed to the closeness of a very specific thing. To some, they may see just a close up of a lime in a glass and wonder to themselves why it's such a big deal to someone like me. That's why there exists an autism spectrum---we simply don't perceive things the way "normal" people do, and that's precisely why I'm sharing this book with everyone.

Lastly, there is very little order to the placements of these photos. There are common themes, but I randomly placed them in each page on purpose. I chose not to caption any of them because I think that would be TELLING instead of SHOWING.

If you can see the same squares, polygons, intersecting lines, ovals, half-circles, and… that I see, then you understand a little bit more this type of autistic mind. You, too, can see as some of us see---in pictures and shapes.

In this example, most people would see a deck covered in snow with some chairs and a table... and a great deal of trees in the background... with predominant colours of brown and white. I, however, see angles and shapes FIRST before I see anything else or notice any other details. Why is this? I'm a visual person, and I associate all things as shapes before I notice what is filled-in and tend to ignore colour almost entirely unless it's white or black (I am not colour-blind, by the way).

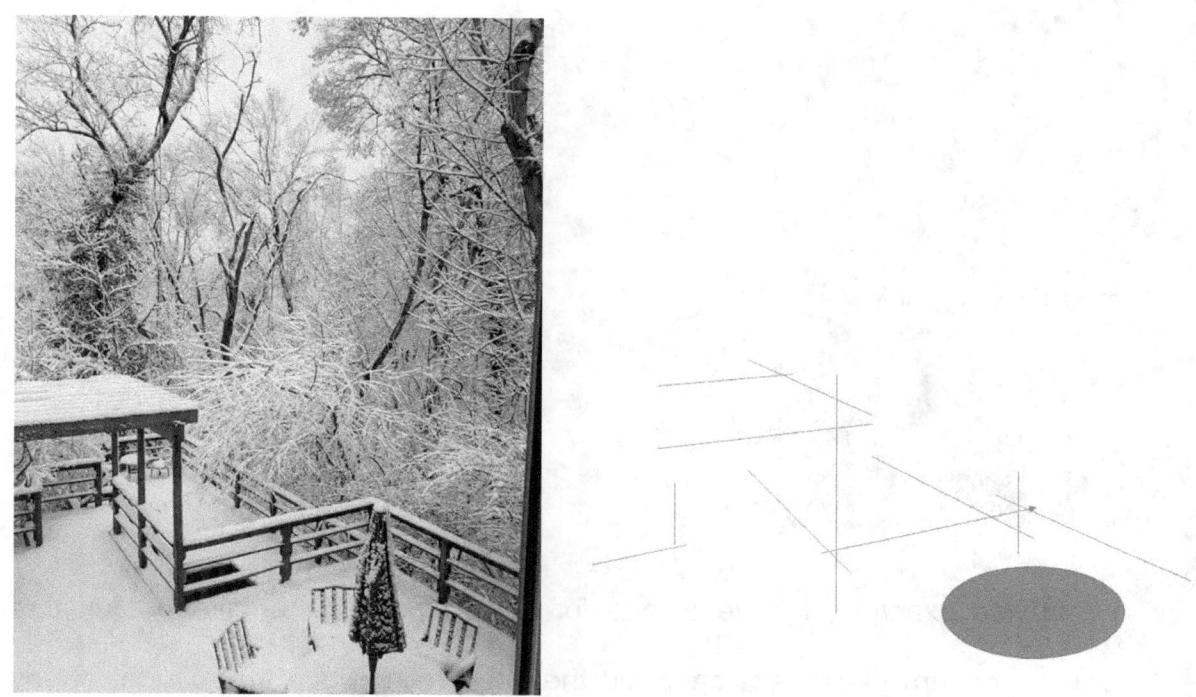

In this example, I took an extreme closeup photo of a water fountain shooting water beneath a ledge. I did not notice the water nor the ledge, at first. I saw intersecting lines that formed shapes (rectangles). Afterward, I noticed the shapes and patterns in-between (the fill-in) then paid attention to the fact it was water and noticed the colours.

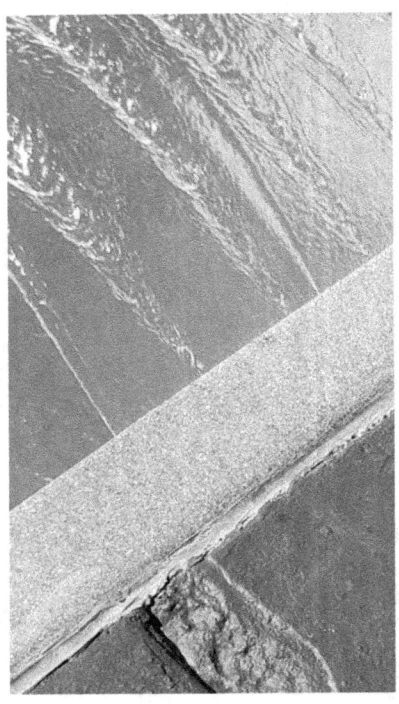 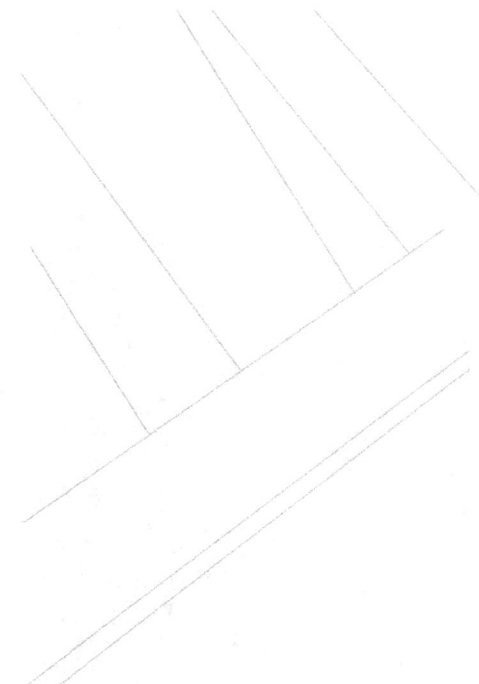

In this example, I have a love for certain brick patterns and took this photo (extreme closeup) because it captured the intersecting lines that caught my eye. If I were asked what colours they were, I would not have been able to recall them---only the shapes.

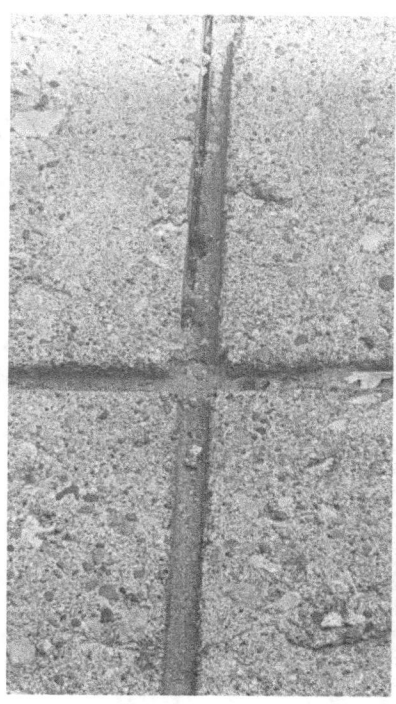

In this final example, I took this photo because I found the intersecting lines to be incredibly beautiful and barely noticed the vegetation growing around it all. If asked about other details, I would be able to recall the colour white and would assume the vegetation was green (by association).

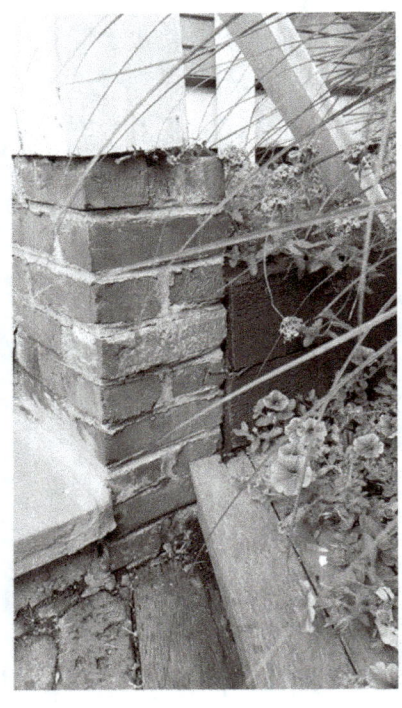
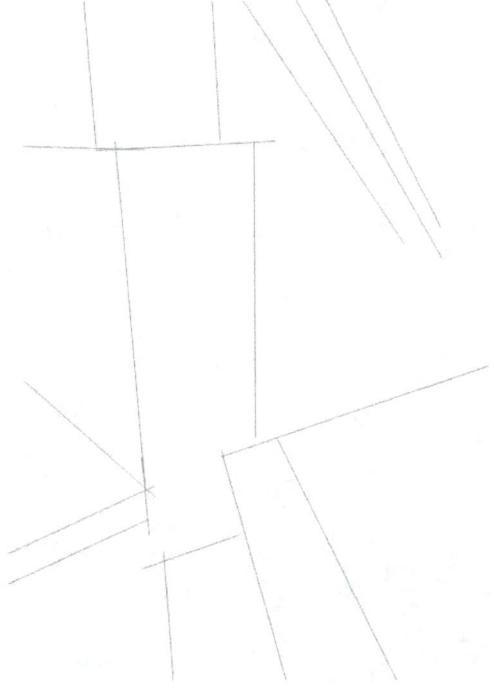

Chapter Conclusion

I highly recommend checking-out my other publication, Patterns in All Things, for a very detailed breakdown on how pattern-based thinking works and looks for more information.

WORKS CITED

[1] WechslerTest.com, "About The Wechsler Intelligence Test," WechslerTest.com, [Online]. Available: https://wechslertest.com/about-wechsler-intelligence-test. [Accessed 04 28 2018].

[2] D. R. Henderson, "Psychosomatic Disorders," Patient, 30 12 2016. [Online]. Available: https://patient.info/health/psychosomatic-disorders. [Accessed 6 5 2018].

[3] A. P. Association, American Psychiatric Association: Diagnostic and Statistical Manual of Mental Disorders, Fifth ed., Arlington, VA: American Psychiatric Association, 2013.

[4] A. P. Association, "Diagnostic and Statistical Manual of Mental Disorders (DSM–5)," 19 04 2018. [Online]. Available: https://www.psychiatry.org/psychiatrists/practice/dsm. [Accessed 19 04 2018].

ABOUT THIS WORK

The purpose for writing this book is to help educate those who are---or are not---on The Autism Spectrum. Perhaps, you know someone who may be autistic. Perhaps it's your child? Your partner? Your friend or co-worker? Perhaps, it's yourself, and you would like to know more about the symptoms and the testing process.

Whatever the reason, it is my intent to put my experiences "out there" to help others. Do I believe there is potential for backlash or discrimination of some kind for me having done so? Possibly, but I do believe the benefits far outweigh the risks.

This book is mixed-in with category and chronology. Since the DSM-V (Diagnostic and Statistical Manual of Mental Disorders, Fifth Edition, 2013) breaks-down Autism Spectrum Disorder by very specific categories, I've decided to model each chapter after the major DSM sections, albeit abbreviated in verbiage since their sub-titles tend to be lengthy. Rather than telling my boring life's story in flat chronological order, I've decided to give my categorical examples according to each section in a general chronology---from infancy to current. I also added sub-categories identified as hyper-sensitive and hypo-sensitive as it's important to show that some things are overwhelming while other things are underwhelming or even desirable.

I also included original entries from journals and notes I jotted-down during my diagnosis period. I wanted to gather as much information (the more empirical the better) to back-up my suspicions at the time. They will be noted as "journal item."

My eventual decision to break this entire subject matter into more than one book (series) was not an easy one. I find the social interaction portion to be a boring one compared to the other traits and diagnoses experiences, but one part cannot exist without the other, so I will make this as painless as possible. Nevertheless, I decided to combine the separate books into this single "pane."

My VERY dry sense of humour will be sprinkled throughout this work---either, intentionally or unintentionally. Some things may come across as being negative or sad when they may actually be quite funny to me---and vice-versa.

I will frequently use the phrase "on The Spectrum" to refer to those of us who have been diagnosed with Autism Spectrum Disorder. Since I'm from The States, I have to adhere to the rules of formal diagnosis. In other countries, there may still be a split between High Functioning Autism, Classic Autism, Asperger's Syndrome, PDD-NOS, etc. I was one who, at first, disagreed with the decision to lump it all into one spectrum, but as I learned more about this thing, it occurred to me that they did, in fact, makes things far easier for everyone involved.

You may note that I often use British spelling in some of my words (adding that Oxford 'u'). This is part of what I am. British anything has fascinated me since my early teen years, and I adapted some of their spelling into my own. Teachers always marked it as an error, and I would often point-out that it was not incorrect in The United Kingdom. Rarely, would my argument win him/her over. Understand that I'm intentionally doing it (spelling autocorrect be damned).

I also tend to use ellipsis in my sentences. I type like I talk, essentially, and I talk with broken phrases---pauses. I say three or four words then pause... say three or four words then pause again. As a result, I reflect this in how I type. Again, this is grammatically incorrect but intentional, nonetheless. I aced all of my grammar courses, so if something doesn't look grammatically-correct, there's a high probability I did it intentionally.

Finally, since I'm a highly visual individual, there will be MANY illustrations, photos, diagrams, and other visual examples to accommodate each section---not as much in this particular book, but far more in the others---this particular book is more contextual since it's telling a lifelong story. I'm a strong believer in not only TELLING others about a thing but in SHOWING others about a thing. There are a large number of books "out there" regarding high functioning autism. I want to SHOW what high functioning autism is like rather than just TELL what it is like---or, as my High School Creative Writing teacher once said: "show don't tell."

www.ingramcontent.com/pod-product-compliance
Lightning Source LLC
Chambersburg PA
CBHW081428220526
45466CB00008B/2308